Practical prescribing for musculoskeletal practitioners

Other books from M&K include

Routine Blood Results Explained 3/e
ISBN: 9781905539888

Blood Results in Clinical Practice
ISBN: 9781905539772

Managing Breathlessness in the Community
ISBN: 9781905539734

Working with Children who need Long-term Respiratory Support
ISBN: 9781905539697

Understanding Chronic Kidney Disease: A guide for the non-specialist
ISBN: 9781905539741

Better Patient Feedback, Better Healthcare
ISBN: 9781905539246

Timely Discharge from Hospital
ISBN: 9781905539550

Mentorship in Healthcare
ISBN: 9781905539703

Self Assessment in X-ray Interpretation series

Limbs • Paediatric Trauma • Axial Trauma • MSK Pathology

Practical prescribing for musculoskeletal practitioners

Julie Dawson, Sheena Hennell
and Ruth Sephton

MT

Practical Prescribing for Musculoskeletal Practitioners 2/e
Dr Julie Dawson
Ruth Sephton
Sheena Hennell

ISBN: 9781905539-78-9

First published 2007
2nd (revised) edition) published 2014

British Library Cataloguing in Publication Data
A catalogue record for this book is available from the British Library

Notice

Clinical practice and medical knowledge constantly evolve. Standard safety precautions must be followed, but, as knowledge is broadened by research, changes in practice, treatment and drug therapy may become necessary or appropriate. Readers must check the most current product information provided by the manufacturer of each drug to be administered and verify the dosages and correct administration, as well as contraindications. It is the responsibility of the practitioner, utilising the experience and knowledge of the patient, to determine dosages and the best treatment for each individual patient. Any brands mentioned in this book are as examples only and are not endorsed by the publisher. Neither the publisher nor the authors assume any liability for any injury and/or damage to persons or property arising from this publication.

To contact M&K Publishing write to:
M&K Update Ltd · The Old Bakery · St. John's Street
Keswick · Cumbria CA12 5AS
Tel: 01768 773030 · Fax: 01768 781099
publishing@mkupdate.co.uk
www.mkupdate.co.uk

Designed and typeset by Mary Blood
Printed in Scotland by Bell & Bain Limited, Glasgow

12/15/16

Contents

List of Tables

Foreword

This book is intended to provide prescribing advice for medical and non-medical prescribers caring for adult patients with common musculoskeletal problems. It will be particularly useful for non-medical practitioners, including independent physiotherapy and podiatry prescribers. Reference is made to current prescribing law and accountability, and the principles of safe prescribing are clearly defined. It gives practical prescribing advice for pain control, osteoporosis, gout and disease-modifying anti-rheumatic drugs.

In this second edition of *Practical Prescribing for Musculoskeletal Practitioners*, we have incorporated the National Institute for Health and Care Excellence (NICE) guidance that is relevant to osteoarthritis, chronic low back pain, osteoporosis, rheumatoid arthritis, neuropathic pain and gout. This will help prescribers comply with this guidance, and the weblinks give rapid access to the relevant online documents. For drugs under patent, we have also included weblinks to the relevant online Summary Product Characteristics (SPC). All references have been updated and we have included a list of common proprietary names in the Appendix. We have also included a range of clinical case histories in Chapter 10 so that the reader can practise prescribing and consider salient prescribing issues. These additions make the book extremely relevant to autonomous practitioners who need to know about the evidence base, NICE guidance and rationale for prescribing for patients with musculoskeletal disorders.

Please note that this book does not provide an exhaustive list of side effects. We therefore strongly advise practitioners to check the British National Formulary (BNF) – www.bnf.org/bnf/index.htm – and the Summary of Product Characteristics (SPC) – via www.medicines.org.uk/EMC – for new and all reported side effects, contra-indications and interactions.

Dr Julie Dawson MB ChB, MD, FRCP
Consultant Rheumatologist, St Helens and Knowsley Teaching Hospitals, NHS Trust
Ruth Sephton MSc, MCSP, FMACP
Consultant Musculoskeletal Physiotherapist, 5 Boroughs Partnership NHS Foundation Trust
Sheena Hennell RN, BA Hons, MSc
Commissioning Manager, Wirral Clinical Commissioning Group

Acknowledgements

The authors gratefully thank their reviewers, Dawn Homer, Pippa McCaffrey and Tracey O'Rourke, for their helpful comments and support.

Chapter 1

Non-medical prescribing: the law and accountability

1.1 Prescribing law

Nurses and pharmacists who are suitably qualified independent prescribers may now prescribe from the full British National Formulary (BNF). Radiographers and optometrists may undertake supplementary prescribing. However, it has taken several years to get to this point.

From 1 May 2006, the nurse prescribers' extended formulary was discontinued and qualified nurse independent prescribers (formerly known as extended formulary nurse prescribers) automatically became entitled to prescribe any licensed medicine for any medical condition within their competence.

From 23 April 2012, changes to the Misuse of Drugs Regulations 2001 relating to nurse and pharmacist independent prescribing of controlled drugs (Misuse of Drugs (Amendment No. 2) (England, Wales and Scotland) Regulations 2012 (Statutory Instrument 2012/973)) came into force.

See: www.legislation.gov.uk/uksi/2012/973/pdfs/uksi_20120973_en.pdf

Since then, both nurse independent prescribers and pharmacist independent prescribers have been able to prescribe any controlled drug listed in schedules 2–5 for any medical condition within their competence (except diamorphine, cocaine and dipipanone for addiction).

Physiotherapists and podiatrists have been able to undertake supplementary prescribing since 2005. In August 2013 the government passed legislation allowing appropriately trained physiotherapists and podiatrists in England to act as independent prescribers. Secondary legislation is due to follow in Scotland, Wales and Northern Ireland.

As a result of this, appropriately qualified and annotated physiotherapists and podiatrists will be able to prescribe any licensed medicine, provided it falls within their individual area of competence and respective scopes of practice, which are defined as follows:

- **A physiotherapist independent prescriber may prescribe any licensed medication within national and local guidelines for any condition within their area of expertise and competence within the overarching framework of human movement, performance and function.**
- **A podiatrist independent prescriber can prescribe only those medicines which are relevant to the treatment of disorders affecting the foot, ankle and associated structures, in line with current practice and consistent with published professional guidance.**

Education programmes to deliver training in independent prescribing for physiotherapy and podiatry practitioners are anticipated to begin in January 2014. Podiatrists and physiotherapists who are currently supplementary prescribers will be required to undertake a conversion course to become independent prescribers.

1.2 Guidance and standards

Guidance and standards exist and apply for all health professionals as detailed below.

The Nursing and Midwifery Council (NMC) has produced new standards of proficiency for nurse and midwife prescribers (NMC June 2006).
See: www.nmc-uk.org/Documents/NMC-Publications/NMC-Standards-proficiency-nurse-and-midwife-prescribers.pdf

The Department of Health (DH) has produced guidance entitled 'Improving Patients' Access to Medicines – A Guide to Implementing Nursing and Pharmacist Independent Prescribing within the NHS in England' (DH 2006).

See: http://www.prescribingforsuccess.co.uk/document_uploads/About/DHGuideApril06.pdf

The regulatory body for the General Pharmaceutical Council is responsible for standards of conduct, ethics and performance and for the registration of Independent pharmacist prescribers.

See: http://www.pharmacyregulation.org/standards/conduct-ethics-and-performance

Pharmacists must prescribe in accordance with 'Medicines, Ethics and Practice' published by the Royal Pharmaceutical Society of Great Britain (RPSGB).

See: www.rpharms.com/mep/download-the-mep.asp

Allied health professionals must act in accordance with the Health and Care Professions Council (HCPC) 'Standards of conduct, performance and ethics (2012)'.

See: www.hpc-uk.org/assets/documents/10003B6EStandardsofconduct,performanceandethics.pdf

The HCPC has developed new standards for prescribing which reflect recent changes in legislation (August 2013). The standards apply to chiropodists/podiatrists and physiotherapists who are trained either as supplementary prescribers or as supplementary and independent prescribers. They also apply to radiographers who have completed training to become supplementary prescribers. They set out expectations of education providers delivering training in prescribing and outline the knowledge, understanding and skills expected of a prescriber. The standards can be found on the following link:

http://www.hpc-uk.org/assets/documents/10004160Standardsforprescribing.pdf

The National Prescribing Centre has developed a single generic competency framework for non-medical prescribers, to be used by clinicians as a source of information and as a tool to reflect on practice and identify continuing professional development (CPD) needs.

See: www.npc.co.uk/improving_safety/improving_quality/resources/single_comp_framework.pdf

1.3 Non-medical prescribing definitions

There are two methods of prescribing:

1. **Independent prescribing**
2. **Supplementary prescribing**

Definition of independent prescribing

With independent prescribing, the non-medical prescriber takes responsibility for the clinical assessment of the patient, establishing a diagnosis and the clinical management required. The non-medical practitioner also takes responsibility for prescribing (where necessary) and the appropriateness of any prescription.

Definition of supplementary prescribing

Supplementary prescribing is defined as a voluntary partnership between an independent prescriber (a doctor or dentist) and a supplementary prescriber, to implement an agreed patient-specific clinical management plan (CMP), with the patient's agreement.

Supplementary prescribing allows nurses, pharmacists and allied health professionals who have completed the relevant training, with their employers' approval, to prescribe in a supplementary prescribing partnership.

Following assessment and diagnosis by the independent prescriber and an agreement on the CMP, the supplementary prescriber may prescribe any medicine for the patient that is referred to in a patient-specific CMP, until the next review by the independent prescriber. There is no formulary for supplementary prescribing and no restrictions on the medical conditions that can be managed under these arrangements.

Supplementary prescribing is also a useful mechanism to enable new independent nurse, pharmacist and allied health professional prescribers to develop their expertise and confidence in prescribing or where a team approach to prescribing is clearly appropriate.

Health professionals acting as supplementary prescribers can prescribe any medicines that can be prescribed by an NHS doctor, including controlled drugs and unlicensed medicines, as agreed in the CMP.

Off-licence medicines

Independent prescribers must take full responsibility for their prescribing, and should only prescribe 'off-licence' (i.e. outside the licensed indication) when it is considered best practice to do so.

1.4 Accountability

Accountability is the professional term for responsibility and is defined for non-medical prescribers in the NMC Standards of Proficiency for Nurse and Midwife

Prescribers (May 2006). The NMC may take disciplinary action when a nurse fails to follow guidelines for professional accountability.

Practice Standard 1

This standard is set out in NMC Standards of Proficiency for Nurse and Midwife Prescribers (May 2006):

- You may only prescribe once you have successfully completed an NMC-approved programme and recorded this on the NMC register.
- You may only prescribe from the formulary linked to your recorded qualification and must comply with statutory requirements applicable to your prescribing practice.
- The ability to prescribe is a privilege granted to you by legislation and your employer and should be seen in this light.

Practice Standard 2

This standard is set out in NMC Standards of Proficiency for Nurse and Midwife Prescribers (May 2006):

- You are professionally accountable for your prescribing decisions, including actions and omissions, and cannot delegate this accountability to any other person.
- You must only ever prescribe within your level of experience and competence, acting in accordance with Clause 6 of the NMC Code of Professional Conduct, Standards for Conduct, Performance and Ethics.
- If you move to another area of practice you must consider the requirements of your new role and only ever prescribe within your level of experience and competence.
- In order to prescribe for a patient or client, you must satisfy yourself that you have undertaken a full assessment, including a thorough history, and where possible accessing a full clinical record.
- You are accountable for your decision to prescribe and must prescribe only where you have relevant knowledge of the patient's health and medical history.
- You must ensure a risk assessment has been undertaken in respect of the patient's other current medication and any potential for confusion with other medicines.

The regulatory body for the General Pharmaceutical Council is responsible for standards of conduct, ethics and performance and for the registration of Independent pharmacist prescribers.

See: http://www.pharmacyregulation.org/standards/conduct-ethics-and-performance

Physiotherapists and podiatrists will be required to comply with the necessary standards of prescribing practice once published by the HCPC.

Continuing professional development (CPD)

Prescribers are expected to recognise the importance of (and their responsibility to) maintain up-to-date knowledge of prescribing. Prescribers must comply with their registering body's CPD requirements.

1.5 Vicarious liability

Liability is the legal term for responsibility. If, for example, a practitioner breaches legislation setting out what they can do within their role, this may be deemed a criminal act. Vicarious liability, where the employer takes legal responsibility for the actions of its staff, provides protection for non-medical prescribers (Caulfield 2004). Non-medical prescribing practitioners prescribing in a self-employed capacity must have personal insurance cover, as vicarious liability would not be applicable in this instance/setting.

It is important to read and be aware of your employer's (NHS Trust's) prescribing policy. For example, in some acute Trusts prescribing policies exclude nurses from prescribing cytotoxics. If a nurse were to act outside the boundaries agreed with their employer by prescribing cytotoxics, they would therefore not be covered by vicarious liability and the employer's insurance policy would not pay out. Professional indemnity cover, as provided through Royal College of Nursing (RCN) membership for example, is vital for nurses in extended roles.

Physiotherapists must also be aware of the principle of vicarious liability, whereby an employer is liable for the acts and omissions of an employee. Employers are therefore duty-bound to ensure that all staff are adequately trained and supervised until they can demonstrate competence in, for example, independent prescribing.

Chapter 2

Safe prescribing

2.1 Principles of safe prescribing

The ability to prescribe safely and competently is a fundamental element of patient care. This chapter outlines the principles of prescribing safely for patients.

Safe prescribing can be sub-divided as follows in order to minimise the chance of a medication or prescribing error:

- **Principles of therapeutics**
- **Principles of treatment**
- **Writing the prescription**
- **Monitoring**

According to the National Coordinating Council for Medication Error Reporting and Prevention (2002), a prescribing error can be defined as a preventable action or omission that may contribute to inappropriate or harmful use of a medicine.

2.2 Principles of therapeutics

Prior to prescribing, during your consultation with and assessment of the patient it is important that you:

- **Understand and have a good knowledge of the pharmacology. Weigh up** both the potential benefits and the potential hazards of treatment and understand the reasons for variability in drug response.

- Base your prescribing choice on best evidence.
- Remember that NICE guidance provides prescribing advice for prescribing clinicians, who should be aware of NICE recommendations and implement them where appropriate. In addition, the National Prescribing Centre is now part of NICE, which helps to facilitate improvements in cost-effective prescribing.
- Grade your evidence base. In this book we have used the approach in the box below, which is adapted from that previously used by the Royal College of Physicians and Scottish Intercollegiate Guidelines Network.
- Maintain your continual professional development (CPD) by keeping up to date and involving the patient in the prescribing decision. Patients who are informed and knowledgeable tend to be more compliant and this may improve adherence *(Whiting, Holford & Begg 2002).*

Evidence grades

Grade A: evidence from meta-analysis of randomised controlled trials from at least one well-designed, controlled study using randomisation.

Grade B: evidence from at least one other type of well-designed, quasi-experimental study based on well-designed non-experimental descriptive studies, e.g. comparative studies, correlation studies, case-control studies.

Grade C: evidence from expert committee reports/opinions and/or the clinical experience of authorities.

2.3 Principles of treatment

Prior to prescribing, it is important to consider the following checklists. Table 2.1 will assist you with the prescribing decision; and Table 2.2 will help you with the prescribing process, once the treatment has been chosen.

Table 2.1: Prescribing decision checklist

Assessment and diagnosis.
Consider and discuss with the patient any alternatives to drug therapy.
If, following discussion, the patient wishes to take the drug:
Choose an appropriate drug, making an evidence-based decision.
Check for any allergies.
Are there any co-morbidities to consider?
Are there any contra-indications? (For example, is the patient pregnant or breast-feeding?)
Check for any drug interactions. (Consider concomitant medication.)

Table 2.2: Prescribing process checklist

Choose the appropriate route and dosage.
Discuss any potential side effects with the patient.
Is there a plan to review and monitor the outcome?
Has there been a full and clear discussion with the patient to aid adherence? Document this, where appropriate.
Is there any specific training required for the patient to take their medication correctly (e.g. training to give self-injections)?

2.4 Writing the prescription

When writing the prescription:

- **Ensure the patient details are correct.**

- Use generic drug names (not brand names) and avoid abbreviations.
- Ensure dose, frequency and route of administration are correct and appropriate. Avoid using the term 'as directed' and specify a minimum dose interval for 'as required' directions.
- Ensure the duration of the prescription is confirmed.
- Refer to the British National Formulary (BNF) and Summary of Product Characteristics (SPC).
- Also consider your hospital/primary care prescribing policy and/or formulary.
- Consider NICE and professional body guidance.
- Add your professional status (for example 'nurse independent prescriber') and signature.
- Nurse prescribers need to include a unique identifier, which is normally their NMC PIN. Ensure that your writing is clear and easy to read.

2.5 Monitoring

When monitoring a patient's progress following prescription:

- Advise the patient to report any reaction or side effect to the prescribing clinician/clinic helpline or to their GP or pharmacist.
- Advise the patient to attend for monitoring if required and as per protocol.
- At follow-up appointments, review the indications for continuing to take the drug.
- Liaise and communicate with the patient's General Practitioner (GP), hospital specialist and other relevant parties.

Multidisciplinary/multiprofessional working

With greater integration and breaking down of traditional NHS boundaries, there is an increasing emphasis on multidisciplinary working. Within multidisciplinary teams, the combined contributions of all the members often underpin successful patient management. Sharing information and access to joint documentation is key to multidisciplinary patient care. To fully develop and support non-medical prescribing within specialist teams, and ultimately drive successful non-medical prescribing, multidisciplinary teams need to develop robust joint record keeping, and joint protocols and standards (combined with regular communications and team meetings).

2.6 Adherence to medication

It is good practice for prescribers to involve and support patients in decision-making on their prescriptions, as this encourages adherence to medication. NICE Guideline CG76 provides guidance for practitioners.

See: http://publications.nice.org.uk/medicines-adherence-cg76

Both medical and non-medical prescribers are ideally placed to promote medicines adherence. Any consultation is a potential educational opportunity and it is worth remembering that an informed patient is much more likely to adhere to medication.

A study (Barber *et al.* 2004) has shown that 30% of patients with chronic diseases have missed at least one dose of medication from a new prescription by day 10, some intentionally and others not. Reasons included side effects, concerns and often a need for more information, particularly among those who intentionally chose not to adhere.

Within supplementary prescribing, the clinical management plan (CMP) encourages concordance, which literally means 'agreement and harmony'. In other words, the non-medical prescriber actively encourages the patient to help with the decision-making process and establishes concordance through partnership agreement.

Table 2.3: Definition of terms

Compliance	The degree to which a patient follows medical advice
Adherence	The degree to which a patient takes the prescribed medication
Concordance	A patient and healthcare professional making decisions together about treatment

Case study: focusing on adherence to medication

Background

Mr Jones is a 34-year-old man who has been diagnosed with early-onset rheumatoid arthritis (RA). He was previously fit and well, playing football with his local five-a-side team once a week, and being a committed member of a tennis club. He works as a civil engineer and has a demanding job, often with long hours, and he has been married for two years.

In line with the management protocol used in the rheumatology unit, he commences on methotrexate, 15mg weekly. Over the next six months, he takes his medication as prescribed, following an effective consultation where he was fully involved in the decision-making process and his RA is well controlled.

He and his wife are keen to start a family and after six months he makes the decision not to continue with the methotrexate; however, he does not inform anyone at either the rheumatology unit or his GP's surgery.

Several months later, he presents at the unit with an acute flare of his RA.
At the patient's consultation, the practitioner should:

- **Engage with Mr Jones, providing rapid access to assessment and support.**
- **Establish Mr Jones' frame of reference and preferences and identify gaps in his knowledge.**
- **Re-educate Mr Jones on the principles of RA management and the implications of not receiving treatment. Following this discussion, test Mr Jones' level of understanding with some questions.**
- **Establish Mr Jones' wishes regarding management of the acute flare and long-term management of his RA.**
- **Negotiate the treatment plan and follow-up.**

Empowering the patient to take control and to negotiate treatment of an incurable condition is paramount. Open access for discussion for patients with RA is essential. Good education and support should help patients adhere to drug therapy. Nevertheless, some patients will veer away from an agreed plan and there should therefore be a system in place to deliver non-punitive care, which allows the patient to re-engage, re-focus and move forward.

See: http://publications.nice.org.uk/medicines-adherence-cg76

Chapter 3

Analgesics

3.1 Overview

Assessing the patient and establishing the cause of their musculoskeletal pain is fundamental to prescribing appropriate medication. Pain can be defined as an unpleasant feeling which may be associated with actual or potential tissue damage and which may have physical and emotional components. It is important to distinguish between pain and nociception. Nociception is a neurophysiological term and refers to specific activity in nerve pathways. Nociception is the transmission mechanism for physiological pain and does not incorporate emotional or central sensitisation components.

When considering all medication treatment options, it is useful to identify whether the patient's pain has one or more of four components:

- **Mechanical nociceptive**
- **Inflammatory nociceptive**
- **Neuropathic**
- **Central sensitisation (Meeus & Nijs 2007)**

In Chapter 4 we will discuss atypical analgesics for pain with a significant neuropathic or central sensitisation component.

When prescribing for pain, you should use the World Health Organisation (WHO) pain management ladder. The analgesic ladder for nociceptive pain basically outlines a stepped change of analgesics, starting with non-opioid, moving to weak opioid and then strong opioid (see Table 3.1 below). With non-opioid and weak opioid, there is usually a ceiling dose. Once the patient is being treated with strong opioid, the dose can be titrated according to the patient's pain and no ceiling dosage is defined.

Table 3.1: Analgesic ladder

Analgesic ladder	Group	Examples described in this chapter
Step 1	Non-opioid NSAID +/- atypical analgesic	Paracetamol see Chapter 4 see Chapter 6
Step 2	Weak opioid +/- non-opioid +/- atypical analgesic	Codeine, tramadol paracetamol, see Chapter 6
Step 3	Strong opioid +/- non-opioid +/- atypical analgesic	Morphine, oxycodone, fentanyl, buprenorphine, tramadol (high dose) paracetamol, NSAID see Chapter 4 see Chapter 6

When prescribing analgesics for musculoskeletal pain, always make sure the patient has taken the analgesic on a regular (by the clock) basis before moving onto the next step of the analgesic ladder.

Analgesics are more effective in preventing pain than in relieving established pain. For example, if a patient is having daily pain but waits until the pain has become unbearable before taking a painkiller, they will continue to be distressed for a further 20–30 minutes (longer for slow-release preparations) while the tablet is being absorbed and transferred to their bloodstream. In this situation, the opportunity for an analgesic to work is greatly diminished and the emotional component of pain is increased. The patient may therefore quickly move up the analgesic ladder, suffering more side effects from medication (such as drowsiness and constipation) and then deciding the tablets have severe side effects that outweigh their benefits.

Medication overuse headaches

These can occur in patients with chronic (three months or more) use of analgesics. Headaches occur when analgesic levels trough – for example, the patient may wake up with a headache in the morning. It is thought that pain-signalling mechanisms become more sensitive with constant suppression by pain-killing medication. NICE have included this in their headache guidance.

See: http://publications.nice.org.uk/headaches-cg150/guidance

They advise practitioners to consider analgesic headache if patients have been taking:

- Opioids
- Combination analgesic medications on 10 days per month or more
- Paracetamol, aspirin or an NSAID, either alone or in any combination, on 15 days per month or more.

All analgesics can cause this problem and it is important to educate patients so that they are aware of this possible effect. This may be sufficient to make them decide to avoid taking further analgesics for the headache. However, with significant symptoms, analgesics may need to be gradually withdrawn to treat the headache, and this may need specialist referral.

3.2 Non-opioid – Step 1

Paracetamol (Acetominophen)

This is a key non-opioid analgesic component of each step of the WHO pain ladder. It is also effective at controlling a fever. It is generally well tolerated with few side effects.

Mechanism of action

Currently thought to be through inhibiting prostaglandins in the brain, resulting in raising the pain threshold.

Evidence grading

Grade A evidence for acute and chronic pain (osteoarthritis) (Toms *et al.* 2008; Towheed *et al.* 2006)

NICE guidance weblink

Low back pain: http://guidance.nice.org.uk/CG88

Preparations

Tablets (500mg), soluble tablets (500mg), oral suspension (120mg/5ml, 250mg/5ml), suppositories (250mg, 500mg)

Dosage

0.5–1.0g, every 4–6 hours (maximum adult dosage: 4g [8 x 500mg tablets] per day/24-hour period)

Side effects

Medication overuse headache.

Relative cautions

Liver disease and severe renal impairment.

Contra-indications

Known hypersensitivity to paracetamol.

Interactions

- The speed of absorption of paracetamol may be increased by metoclopramide or domperidone.
- Delayed absorption by colestyramine.
- Prolonged regular intake may increase the risk of bleeding for patients on warfarin or coumarins.
- Increased plasma concentration of chloramphenicol.

Prescribing advice

Paracetamol should be tried on a regular 1g (four times a day) regime prior to prescribing additional medication. Regular paracetamol is the first-line medication treatment option advised in the NICE Low Back Pain Guidance .

Caution all patients against taking more than eight tablets per day/24-hour period. Serious liver damage can occur with only small increases above the normal limit (e.g. 5g per day) in susceptible individuals. It is not always possible to predict who is at high risk of susceptibility to liver damage. Two groups of patients with high susceptibility are those that are:

- **At risk of cytochrome P450 induction due to excess alcohol intake or medication (e.g. phenytoin, phenobarbitone, carbamazepine, rifampicin, St John's Wort)**
- **Those that have glutathione depletion (e.g. from starvation, cystic fibrosis, HIV infection).**

Recent publications have raised the possibility that long-term full dosage paracetamol ingestion was associated with liver enzyme abnormalities. Transient increases in alanine transaminases have been reported, but these have not deteriorated into liver failure when maximum daily doses are avoided (Kuffner *et al.* 2006, Watkins *et al.* 2006).

3.3 Weak opioid – Step 2

Codeine

Most prescribing formularies will suggest codeine as the first line to try on the second step of the analgesic ladder. Weak opioids are often combined with paracetamol. If the paracetamol dose (see above) is limiting the dose of opioid in a combination tablet, consider prescribing the opioid and paracetamol separately.

Mechanism of action

Codeine is metabolised in the body, by an enzyme process called demethylation, to morphine. Only 10% of the compound is converted to morphine. This then stimulates the opioid (mu and kappa) receptors in the central nervous system, causing inhibition of the spinal and central processing of pain sensation.

Evidence grading

Grade A evidence for acute and chronic pain (de Craen *et al.* 1996; Furlan *et al.* 2006; Moore *et al.* 2011a; Toms *et al.* 2009)

NICE guidance weblinks

Osteoarthritis: http://guidance.nice.org.uk/CG59
Low back pain: http://guidance.nice.org.uk/CG88

Preparations

Tablets (15mg, 30mg, 60mg), syrup (25mg/5ml)

- Codeine combined with paracetamol available as tablet, dispersible or effervescent tablets or capsules in the following strengths: co-codamol 8/500 = 8mg codeine/500mg paracetamol

- co-codamol 15/500 = 15mg codeine/500mg paracetamol
- co-codamol 30/500 = 30mg codeine/500mg paracetamol

Dosage

30–60mg, every 4–6 hours (maximum dosage: 240g per day)

Side effects

Commonly nausea, vomiting, constipation, dizziness, sweating, dependence, medication overuse headache.

Relative cautions

Use as low a dose as possible in the elderly, and patients with hypothyroidism, hypoadrenalism, chronic hepatic disease and renal insufficiency. As codeine may cause the release of histamine, it should be given with caution to asthmatics. Caution is also advised with patients who are pregnant or breastfeeding.

Contra-indications

Known hypersensitivity to any of the tablet constituents; respiratory depression; obstructive airways disease; paralytic ileus; head injury; raised intracranial pressure; acute alcoholism. As codeine may cause the release of histamine, it should not be given during an asthma attack.

Interactions

- Other central nervous system depressants, including sedatives, phenothiazines, and alcohol, may result in respiratory depression or sedation.
- Monoamine oxidase inhibitors (MAOIs) or within two weeks of such therapy-enhanced sedative effect of codeine or anti-depressant effect of MAOI.
- Mexiletine – codeine delays absorption.
- Codeine antagonises effects of domperidone and metoclopramide on gastro-intestinal activity.
- Cimetidine inhibits the metabolism of opioid analgesics, resulting in increased plasma concentrations of opioid.

Prescribing advice

The amount of codeine in combined preparations varies. It is important to be aware of the different dosages and combinations available, and try to match them according to the required control of pain and the side effects the patients are prone to.

The conversion of codeine to morphine occurs in the liver and is catalysed by the cytochrome P450 enzyme CYP2D6. Approximately 6–10% of the Caucasian population have poorly functional CYP2D6 and codeine is therefore not effective as an analgesic in these patients but they still have its side effects (Eckhardt *et al.* 1998). Dependence can occur after a short period of treatment, and withdrawal symptoms may develop on stopping the drug.

Tramadol

Use when codeine is ineffective or troublesome because of constipation. Tramadol may have less respiratory depression and be possibly less addictive than codeine. It can be effective in managing neuropathic pain, and is a third-line treatment recommendation in the NICE guidance 'Neuropathic pain – pharmacological management CG96' (2010).

Mechanism of action

Tramadol's analgesic properties are thought to derive from the binding of sigma, kappa, mu-opioid receptors, inhibition of noradrenaline reuptake, and serotonin release.

Evidence grading

Grade A evidence for chronic and neuropathic pain (Cepeda *et al.* 2006; Deshpande *et al.* 2007; Duehmke, Hollingshead & Cornblath 2006; Manchikanti *et al.* 2011).

NICE guidance weblinks

Osteoarthritis:http://guidance.nice.org.uk/CG59
Low back pain: http://guidance.nice.org.uk/CG88
Neuropathic pain: http://guidance.nice.org.uk/CG96

Preparations

- Capsules (50mg), orodispersible tablets (50mg) or soluble tablets (50mg)
- Modified release tablets, twice-daily regime (100mg, 150mg, 200mg tablets)
- Modified release tablets, once-daily regime (100mg, 150mg, 200mg, 300mg, 400mg)
- Modified release capsules, twice-daily regime (50mg, 100mg, 150mg, 200mg)

Tramadol combined with paracetamol is 37.5mg tramadol with 325mg paracetamol tablets.

Dosage

- 50–100mg, not more often than 4-hourly
- Modified release, twice-daily preparations: initially 50–100mg twice daily
- Once-daily tablets: initially 100mg or 150mg daily (maximum dosage: 400mg per day)

Side effects

In addition to those side effects experienced with codeine, nausea and vomiting are more common. Abdominal discomfort, hypotension, psychiatric disturbance (hallucinations), convulsions can also occur.

Interactions

- Other central nervous system depressants, including sedatives, phenothiazines, and alcohol, may result in respiratory depression or sedation.
- Monoamine oxidase inhibitors (MAOIs) or within two weeks of such therapy enhanced sedative effect of tramadol or anti-depressant effect of MAOIs.
- May increase the potential for other seizure threshold-lowering drugs to cause convulsions, examples being selective serotonin re-uptake inhibitors (SSRIs), tricyclic anti-depressants (TCAs), and anti-psychotics.
- Rarely, cases of serotonergic syndrome have been reported with the therapeutic use of tramadol in combination with other serotonergic agents such as SSRIs.
- Carbamazepine results in markedly decreased serum concentrations of tramadol, which may reduce analgesic effectiveness and shorten the duration of action.
- Warfarin and coumarin may cause increased international normalised ratio (INR) and bruising in some patients.
- The combination of mixed agonists/antagonists (e.g. buprenorphine, nalbuphine, pentazocine) and tramadol is not recommended because it is theoretically possible that the analgesic effect of a pure agonist will be attenuated under these circumstances.

Contra-indications

As for codeine: known hypersensitivity to any of the tablet constituents; respiratory depression; obstructive airways disease; paralytic ileus; head injury; raised intracranial pressure; acute alcoholism. Also, patients with uncontrolled epilepsy, pregnancy and breastfeeding.

Prescribing advice

For those patients taking 4- to 6-hourly regular doses of tramadol, consider changing to the modified release preparations. However, in patients over 75 years of age with liver and renal impairment, and for patients with serious renal or hepatic impairment, modified release preparations are not recommended, as prolonged elimination occurs.

If patients are intolerant of tramadol, a possible alternative is Tramacet®.

See: www.medicines.org.uk/EMC/medicine/22196/SPC

This may have equal potency to tramadol by combining tramadol and paracetamol, but the lower tramadol dose results in an improved side effect profile. It has also been shown to be effective in controlling the pain of fibromyalgia when compared to placebo (Bennett *et al.* 2003).

3.4 Strong opioid – Step 3

The strong opioids most commonly used for chronic musculoskeletal nociceptive pain in the UK are morphine, oxycodone, fentanyl and buprenorphine, and these are considered below. Use only if you are familiar with, and according to, the British Pain Society's 'Opioids for persistent pain: Good Practice' (2010).

See: www.britishpainsociety.org/book_opioid_main.pdf

The use of strong opioids as modified release preparations is the preferred option for patients with persistent pain (British Pain Society 2010). If pain relief is not achieved with the equivalent of 120–180mg morphine per day, referral to a Specialist in Pain Medicine is strongly recommended.

Morphine

Morphine is considered the first-choice strong opioid in most hospital formularies for chronic non-malignant pain. However, many patients find it difficult to accept this medication because of the strong public perception that morphine is associated with cancer, death and addiction.

Mechanism of action

Morphine's effects are thought to be from agonism of mu opiate receptor, with a smaller contribution from agonism of the kappa opiate receptor.

Evidence grading

Grade A evidence for chronic pain and neuropathic pain (Eisenberg, McNicol & Carr 2006; Furlan *et al.* 2006; Noble *et al.* 2010).

Preparations

- Oral solution (as 10mg/5ml, 30mg/5ml and 100mg/5ml)
- Tablets (10mg, 20mg, 50mg)
- Suppositories (10mg, 15mg, 20mg, 30mg)
- Injections (10, 15, 20 and 30mg/ml)
- Modified release oral preparations – see Dosage (below).

Dosage

No ceiling dose. (See also Prescribing advice, page 23.)

To be taken every 12 hours:

- Tablets (5mg, 10mg, 15mg, 30mg, 60mg, 100mg, 200mg)
- Suspension (20mg, 30mg, 60mg, 100mg, 200mg)
- Capsules (10mg, 30mg, 60mg, 100mg, 200mg)

To be taken every 24 hours:

- Capsules (30mg, 60mg, 90mg, 120mg, 150mg, 200mg)

Side effects

The major risk of opioid excess is respiratory depression. This can be fatal. The most common side effects at usual doses are nausea, constipation, confusion, occasionally vomiting, and medication overuse headaches. Physical and psychological dependence may appear after taking therapeutic doses for periods of just one to two weeks. Some cases of dependence have been observed after only two to three days. Withdrawal syndrome (nausea, vomiting, diarrhoea, anxiety and shivering) may occur a few hours after withdrawal of a prolonged treatment, and is maximal between the 36th and 72nd hours.

Cautions

Use as low a dose as possible in the elderly, and patients with hypothyroidism, hypoadrenalism, chronic hepatic disease, renal insufficiency, hypotension, epilepsy, asthma and prostatic hypertrophy.

Contra-indications

Known hypersensitivity to any of the tablet constituents; respiratory depression;

obstructive airways disease; paralytic ileus; head injury; raised intracranial pressure; acute alcoholic intoxication and delirium tremens. Pregnancy and breastfeeding.

Interactions

- Other central nervous system depressants, including sedatives, phenothiazines, and alcohol, may result in respiratory depression or sedation.
- Monoamine oxidase inhibitors (MAOIs) or within two weeks of MAOI therapy, enhanced sedative effect of opioid or anti-depressant effect of MAOI.
- Cyclizine may counteract the haemodynamic benefits of opioids.
- Opioid analgesics with some antagonist activity, such as buprenorphine, nalbuphine or pentazocine, may precipitate withdrawal symptoms in patients who have recently used pure agonists such as morphine.
- Mexiletine-concomitant opioid use delays its absorption.
- Antagonises effects of domperidone and metoclopramide on the gastrointestinal activity.

Prescribing advice

Only prescribe opiates if you are aware of the British Pain Society's 'Opioids for persistent pain: Good Practice' (2010), and this treatment has been fully discussed with the patient and regular follow-up of the patient can be provided.

It must be emphasised that this is only a guide to the dose of strong opioid required. Inter-patient variability requires that each patient should be carefully titrated to the appropriate dose. Patients should be closely monitored after any change in medication, and titration of dose is to be expected. Patients and relatives need readily accessible support.

Start with 5–10mg of morphine, or 10–20mg if full dosage Step 2 analgesics have been used previously. Halve the dose in elderly patients or if there is a co-morbidity as described above. Give a short-acting (4-hourly) preparation and adjust the dose according to the pain. Once the pain is controlled, the patient's 24-hourly morphine requirement can be determined, and this can then be given as two divided doses (12-hourly regime) or as a single once-daily dose.

During the first week of morphine treatment, troublesome nausea and vomiting is to be expected so co-prescribe an antiemetic as a routine. Domperidone (10mg three times a day), haloperidol (0.5micrograms at night), ondansetron (unlicensed indication) are most commonly used. Constipation is also so predictable that an adjuvant laxative should be prescribed. Around 80% of patients prescribed strong opiates develop at least one side effect. Explain this before commencing treatment and document each side effect on follow-up (British Pain Society 2010).

Oxycodone

Oxycodone is a semi-synthetic pharmacologically active full opioid agonist. It may cause more constipation than morphine but less nausea and hallucinations. It has a rapid onset of action.

Mechanism of action

It is a mu, kappa and delta opioid receptor agonist. It has no antagonist properties. It does not require conversion to oxymorphine to be effective.

Evidence grading

Grade A evidence for acute and chronic pain (Furlan *et al.* 2006; Moore *et al.* 2011a).

Preparations

- Capsules (5mg, 10mg, 20mg)
- Liquid (5mg/5ml)
- Concentrate (10mg/ml)
- Injection (10mg/ml)
- Modified release tablets (5mg, 10mg, 20mg, 40mg, 80mg) to be taken 12-hourly

Dosage

No ceiling dose. For chronic non-malignant pain, 40mg per day is the average dose to control symptoms.

Side effects

As for morphine (see page 22).

Relative cautions

Adults with mild to moderate renal impairment and mild hepatic impairment. Halve the initial starting dose for opioid-naive patients.

Contra-indications

As for morphine (see page 22), severe hepatic and renal impairment (creatinine clearance <10ml/min).

Interactions

- Other central nervous system depressants, including sedatives, phenothiazines, and alcohol, may result in respiratory depression or sedation.
- Monoamine oxidase inhibitors (MAOIs) or, within two weeks of such therapy, enhanced sedative effect of opioid or anti-depressant effect of MAOI.
- Inhibitors of cytochrome P450 (e.g. quinidine, cimetidine, ketoconazole, erythromycin), may inhibit metabolism of oxycodone.

Prescribing advice

The usual starting dose for opioid-naive patients, or patients presenting with severe pain uncontrolled by weaker opioids, is 5mg, 4- to 6-hourly. The dose should then be carefully titrated (as frequently as once a day if necessary) to achieve pain relief.

Patients receiving oral morphine before oxycodone therapy should have their daily dose based on the following ratio: 10mg of oral oxycodone is equivalent to 20mg of oral morphine.

Fentanyl

Fentanyl is 80 times more potent than morphine and can only be used in opioid-tolerant patients. It is probably less constipating than morphine. Only fentanyl, as patches, is licensed for chronic non-malignant pain.

Mechanism of action

A synthetic opioid with high affinity for the mu-opioid receptor.

Evidence grading

Grade A evidence for chronic pain (Langford *et al.* 2006; van Ojik *et al.* 2012).

Preparations

Patches:

- '12' (releasing approx. 12 micrograms/hour for 72 hours)
- '25' (releasing approx. 25 micrograms/hour for 72 hours)
- '50' (releasing approx. 50 micrograms/hour for 72 hours)
- '75' (releasing approx. 75 micrograms/hour for 72 hours)
- '100' (releasing approx. 100 micrograms/hour for 72 hours)

Dosage

Start at '25' patch in patients who are on full dosage of weak opioids. In those already receiving strong opioid, 90mg of oral morphine over 24 hours is approximately equivalent to 25 micrograms/hour fentanyl patch.

A conversion table is available on the electronic medicines compendium website. **See: www.medicines.org.uk/EMC/medicine/17086/SPC**

As the serum levels gradually increase after applying the patch, allow at least 24 hours of treatment before changing dose. At 300 micrograms/hour, alternative pain treatment should be considered.

Side effects

The most serious adverse reaction, as with all potent opioids, is respiratory suppression. Other opioid-related adverse reactions include: nausea; vomiting; constipation; hypotension; bradycardia; somnolence; headache; confusion; hallucinations; euphoria; pruritus; sweating and urinary retention. Involuntary muscle contractions can occur. Skin reactions such as rash, erythema and itching have occasionally been reported. These reactions usually resolve within 24 hours of removal of the patch. Opioid withdrawal symptoms may occur in some patients after changing from their previous analgesic to fentanyl patches.

Cautions

Bradyarrhythmias, chronic respiratory disease, raised intracranial pressure, elderly, significant liver and renal disease, and fever (increased absorption from patch).

Contra-indications

As for morphine (see page 22).

Interactions

- Other central nervous system depressants, including sedatives, phenothiazines, and alcohol, may result in respiratory depression or sedation.
- Monoamine oxidase inhibitors (MAOIs) or, within two weeks of such therapy, enhanced sedative effect of opioid or anti-depressant effect of MAOI. With cytochrome P450 3A4 inhibitors (e.g. ritonavir, ketoconazole, itraconazole, clarithromycin, erythromycin, nelfinavir, verapamil, diltiazem and amiodarone), may result in an increase in fentanyl plasma concentrations.

Prescribing advice

The patient should have had full dosage of a weak opioid before transfer to patch. See morphine prescribing advice (page 23). Titrate the dose up by adding fentanyl

'12' patch. Routinely prescribe an anti-emetic for the first week of treatment. Evaluation of pain control should not be made for at least 24 hours after the patch has been applied, and the dose should be adjusted at 48–72 hours.

The patch should be applied to a clean, dry, non-irritated, non-hairy flat area of the upper arm or body. The transdermal patch should be pressed firmly in place for approximately 30 seconds, making sure the contact is complete, especially around the edges. When changing to a new patch, it should be applied to a different skin site. Advise the patient to wait several days before a new patch is applied to the same area of skin.

Heat, whether internal (such as a fever) or external (such as a sauna), can potentially increase fentanyl delivery rate. It is therefore necessary to avoid exposure to external heat, or monitor for opioid side effects if there is a significant increase in body temperature. It may take 22 hours or longer for plasma fentanyl levels to decrease by 50% when a patch is removed and not replaced. Alternative opioid treatment should be initiated at a low dose and titrated slowly.

Buprenorphine

This drug is a mixed agonist/antagonist used for moderate to severe pain. It is not administered orally, due to very high first pass metabolism. Opiate antagonist effects are not usually seen when combined with weak opioid. However, buprenorphine can precipitate withdrawal symptoms in patients who are physically dependent on full agonist opiates. Its effects can only be partially blocked by naloxone.

Mechanism of action

Synthetic opioid, partially stimulates the mu-opioid receptors, kappa-opioid receptor antagonist.

Evidence grading

Grade A evidence for chronic pain (van Ojik *et al.* 2012; Sorge & Sittl 2004; Steiner *et al.* 2011)

Preparation

Once-weekly transdermal patches:

- '5' (releasing 5 micrograms/hour for 7 days
- '10' (releasing 10 micrograms/hour for 7 days)
- '20' (releasing 20 micrograms/hour for 7 days)

Twice-weekly transdermal patches:

- '35' (releasing 35 micrograms/hour for 96 hours)
- '52.5' (releasing 52.5 micrograms/hour for 96 hours)
- '70' (releasing 70 micrograms/hour for 96 hours)

Sublingual tablets: 200 and 400 micrograms

Dosage

Patches (see Prescribing advice below)

Sublingual tablets: 200–400 micrograms every 8 hours

Side effects

Similar to those of other opioids and include nausea and vomiting, drowsiness, dizziness, headache, itch, dry mouth, miosis, orthostatic hypotension, male ejaculatory difficulty, decreased libido, urinary retention, constipation, physical and psychological dependence. Local reactions to the patches are common.

Cautions

Convulsive disorders, head injury, reduced level of consciousness of uncertain origin, intra-cranial lesions or increased intra-cranial pressure. Patients with severe hepatic impairment.

Contra-indications

Hypersensitivity to any of the excipients; conditions in which the respiratory centre and function are severely impaired or may become so; patients suffering from myasthenia gravis or delirium tremens. Pregnancy and breast-feeding.

Interactions

- Other central nervous system depressants, including sedatives, phenothiazines, and alcohol, may result in respiratory depression or sedation.
- Monoamine oxidase inhibitors (MAOIs) or, within two weeks of such therapy, enhanced sedative effect of opioid or anti-depressant effect of MAOI. Strong opioid – may precipitate withdrawal symptoms.
- If administered together with inhibitors of P450 CYP 3A4 (e.g. ritonavir, ketoconazole, itraconazole, clarithromycin, erythromycin, nelfinavir, verapamil, diltiazem and amiodarone), the buprenorphine plasma levels may be increased.

Prescribing advice

Patients do not need to be on full dosage of a weak opioid to convert to weekly buprenorphine patches. However, with the more potent 96-hour patches, prior experience of reasonable doses of weak opioids is recommended. Patients who have not received any analgesia or have received non-opioids or weak opioids should be started on '35' patch. For patients receiving more than 120mg of oral morphine/day, it is recommended in the SPC that a 52.5 micrograms/hour patch is used first.

See: www.medicines.org.uk/EMC/medicine/8864/SPC

Clearly, it is of major concern that the narcotic effects of overdose cannot be completely reversed by naloxone, and buprenorphine should be avoided in patients thought to be at risk of overdosing (either deliberately or inadvertently).

The patch should be applied to a clean, dry, non-irritated, non-hairy flat area of the upper arm or body. The transdermal patch should be pressed firmly in place for approximately 30 seconds, making sure the contact is complete, especially around the edges. When changing patches, the old patch should be removed gently and the new patch should then be applied to a different skin site. Advise the patient to wait several days before a new patch is applied to the same area of skin. If these precautions are not followed, some patients may experience an allergic reaction to the adhesive used in these patches, which may prevent their continued use.

Heat, whether internal (such as a fever) or external (such as a sauna), can potentially increase buprenorphine delivery rate. It is therefore necessary to avoid exposure to external heat, or monitor for opioid side effects if there is a significant increase in body temperature. It may take 24 hours or longer for plasma buprenorphine levels to decrease by 50% when a patch is removed and not replaced. Alternative opioid treatment should be avoided for 24 hours after removing the patch if possible.

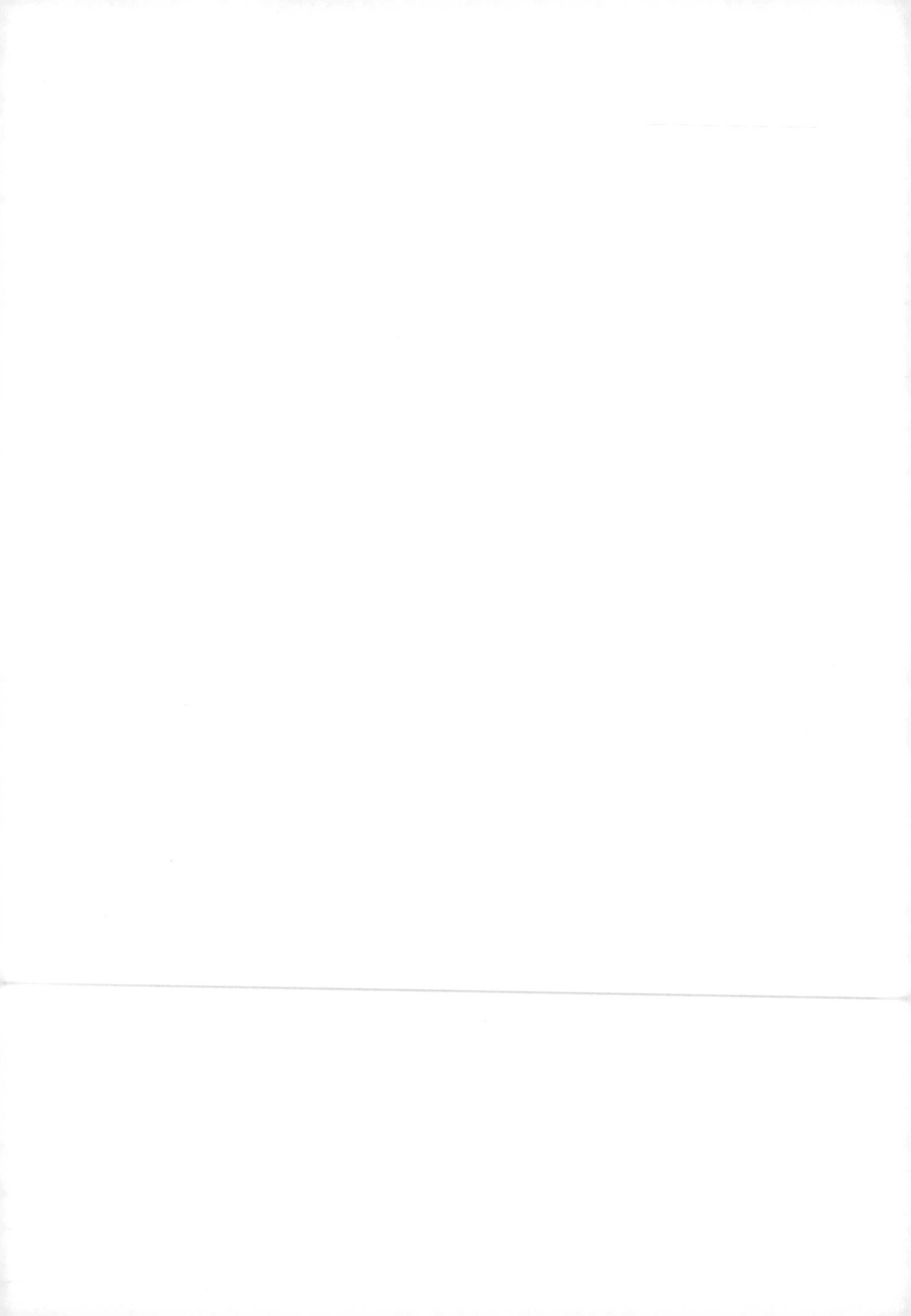

Chapter 4

Atypical analgesics

4.1 Overview

These are medications that are effective for pain but do not utilise the opiate receptor pathway. They are usually for neuropathic pain or have been demonstrated to be of help in chronic pain syndromes such as fibromyalgia. These medicines were originally introduced for the treatment of depression or epilepsy. Now they are being designed specifically to treat neuropathic pain.

Neuropathic pain is spontaneous pain that is frequently described as 'shooting', 'burning' or 'electric shock-like'. Patients frequently find it impossible to describe. Often it is associated with symptoms such as numbness and pins and needles. Signs are hyperalgesia (increased sensation of pain in response to normally painful stimuli) and allodynia (pain in response to normally non-painful stimuli).

The NICE guidance 'Neuropathic pain – pharmacological management CG96' (2010) recommends pregabalin or amitriptyline first line for non-diabetic neuropathic pain, and duloxetine or amitriptyline first line for painful diabetic neuropathy. Tramadol (described in Chapter 3, page 19) and topical lidocaine are third-line treatment options for neuropathic pain.

4.2 Amitriptyline, nortriptyline and imipramine

Although widely used for neuropathic pain, and where there is significant sleep disturbance associated with chronic pain, these drugs are not actually licensed for pain.

Amitriptyline is recommended as a first-line treatment for non-diabetic neuropathic pain from any cause in the NICE neuropathic pain guidance (2010), and tricyclic anti-depressants are recommended for use in the NICE low back pain guidance (2009), when other medications are insufficient to manage the patient's pain. They are licensed as anti-depressants and for nocturnal enuresis and not for pain relief.

Nortriptyline is the principal active metabolite of amitriptyline and seems to have fewer side effects, although tachycardia can be troublesome. Imipramine is suggested as an alternative to try in the NICE neuropathic pain guidance if amitriptyline has been ineffective. This is based on pharmacological evidence that individual patients react very differently to tricyclic anti-depressants, and failure with one tricyclic anti-depressant does not necessarily predict failure with another.

Mechanism of action

The precise mechanism of action is unknown. These drugs have anti-cholinergic and sedative properties, and prevent the re-uptake of noradrenaline and serotonin at nerve terminals.

Evidence grading

Grade A evidence for chronic pain (fibromyalgia) and neuropathic pain (Häuser *et al.* 2012; McQuay, Carroll, & Glynn 1992; Moore *et al.* 2012; Saarto & Wiffen 2007)

NICE guidance weblinks

Low back pain: http://guidance.nice.org.uk/CG88
Neuropathic pain: http://guidance.nice.org.uk/CG96

Preparations

- Amitriptyline tablets (10mg, 25mg, 50mg)
- Amitriptyline oral solution (25mg/5ml, 50mg/5ml)
- Nortriptyline tablets (10mg, 25mg)
- Imipramine tablets (10mg, 25mg)
- Imipramine oral solution (25mg/5ml)

Dosage

Usually 10–75mg nocte. Use as low a dose as possible in elderly and adolescent patients.

Side effects

Drowsiness, dizziness, postural hypotension, nausea, constipation, blurred vision, dry mouth, difficulty with micturition, sinus tachycardia, agitation, hyponatraemia. Lowered seizure threshold.

Caution

Epilepsy, closed angle glaucoma, liver disease, cardiac disease, thyrotoxicosis, psychoses, prostatic hypertrophy or urinary retention, porphyria.

Contra-indications

Hypersensitivity to amitriptyline, nortriptyline or imipramine, recent myocardial infarction and arrhythmias, pregnancy and breast-feeding.

Interactions

- Monoamine oxidase inhibitors (MAOIs) or, within three weeks of such therapy, enhanced sedative effect of opioid or anti-depressant effect of MAOI. There is a risk of MAOI crisis, leading to severe symptoms such as hypertensive crisis, hyperpyrexia, myoclonus, agitation, seizures, delirium and coma.
- Sympathomimetic drugs (such as adrenaline/epinephrine, ephedrine, isoprenaline, noradrenaline/norepinephrine, phenylephrine and phenylpropanolamine) potentiate the cardiovascular effects.
- Guanethidine, bethanidine and clonidine decrease the anti-hypertensive effect of adrenergic neurone blockers.
- Barbiturates may increase the rate of metabolism of these drugs.
- Anaesthetics given during tricyclic anti-depressant therapy may increase the risk of arrhythmias and hypotension.
- Other central nervous system depressants, including sedatives, phenothiazines, and alcohol, may result in sedation.
- Higher than expected steady-state serum concentrations of the tricyclic anti-depressant have been observed when therapy is initiated in patients who are already taking cimetidine. A decrease may occur when cimetidine therapy is discontinued.
- Any drug that utilises the hepatic cytochrome P450IID6 isoenzyme system may compete for metabolism by this system, and lead to drug interactions. Lower doses than are usually prescribed for either the tricyclic anti-depressant or the other drug may therefore be required. Examples of drugs that are metabolised by this isoenzyme (including other anti-depressants) are fluoxetine, phenothiazines, carbamazepine, propafenone and flecainide.

- Drugs that inhibit this enzyme (such as quinidine) should be approached with caution.
- Other anti-cholinergic drugs, resulting in increased anti-cholinergic side effects.
- Tricyclic anti-depressants can lower seizure threshold and may antagonise the effect of anti-epileptic drugs.
- Dopaminergic agents: CNS toxicity may be enhanced when tricyclic anti-depressants are co-prescribed with dopaminergic drugs such as selegiline and entacapone.

Prescribing advice

Spend at least 5 minutes explaining to the patient how to take the tablets, their potential side effects and the fact that they are anti-depressants (albeit being used at a much lower dose and as a treatment for pain). This helps improve compliance and avoids unused prescriptions. Remember that these drugs are prescribed 'off label' (unlicensed indication) in this instance. This should be explained to the patient and their consent obtained and documented (NICE back pain guidance 2009).

The effective dose can be anywhere between 10 and 75mg per day. Start with 10mg per day and increase in 10mg increments fortnightly. If it works at a low dose and the patient benefits, they may remain on that dose.

Amitriptyline should be taken 2–4 hours before planned sleep, rather than at bedtime, as this helps to reduce the 'hangover effect' in the morning. Warn the patients about this and also warn them about dizziness and tiredness. Encourage them to keep taking the tablets despite these side effects. With time, they are likely to settle. Discourage them from drinking alcohol whilst taking these tablets. Drivers and people who operate heavy machinery should be advised to be cautious about this side effect. If the 'hangover effect' is significant, they will need to avoid these activities until it settles. It may therefore be best to start the tablets at the weekend.

In susceptible or particularly cautious patients, start with 10mg of nortriptyline and increase in 10mg increments every fortnight.

Advise the patient that these tablets need to be taken regularly to be most effective. Sleep improvement may occur quite quickly but improved pain control can take 2–3 weeks. If patients find the medication helpful, recommend that they continue it for several months. Withdrawal symptoms (such as nausea, headache and dizziness) can occur on suddenly stopping these medications. Whilst these drugs are not addictive, it is best to wean patients off them gradually, rather than stopping them abruptly, in order to minimise withdrawal symptoms.

4.3 Gabapentin

Licensed for neuropathic pain.

Mechanism of action

Gabapentin is similar in structure to the neurotransmitter GABA but is not believed to act on the same brain receptors. Its exact mechanism of action is unknown, but its therapeutic action on neuropathic pain is thought to be due to binding to the alpha2-delta subunit of the voltage-dependent calcium ion channel in the central nervous system, blocking channel action and thus calcium influx.

Evidence grading

Grade A evidence for chronic neuropathic pain and fibromyalgia (Moore *et al.* 2011b).

Preparations

- Capsules (100mg, 300mg, 400mg)
- Tablets (600mg, 800mg)

Dosage

300–1800mg/day. Dose titration is required.

Side effects

The most common side effects are: nausea, dry mouth, arthralgia, dizziness, drowsiness, constipation, loss of appetite, itching skin, sore gums, indigestion, sexual difficulties, restlessness, weight gain, tremor, slurred speech, pain/burning/tingling in the hands/feet, oedema, diarrhoea, flatulence, leucopenia and diplopia. However, gabapentin has an extensive list of common side effects. We therefore suggest looking up any reported side effect on product information (SPC).

Cautions

For the elderly and patients with renal impairment, reduce the dose.

See:www.medicines.org.uk/EMC/medicine/17095/SPC]

Contra-indications

Hypersensitivity to gabapentin. Pregnancy and breast-feeding.

Interactions

- Antacids can reduce absorption so avoid taking for 2 hours after antacid.
- Other central nervous system depressants, including sedatives, phenothiazines, and alcohol, may result in sedation.

Prescribing advice

Gabapentin can be effective for neuropathic pain. However, in general, tricyclic anti-depressants and pregabalin are tolerated better and are more cost effective (NICE neuropathic pain guidance 2010). In patients with central sensitisation of pain, gabapentin can be tried when tricyclic anti-depressants are ineffective, contra-indicated or the patient refuses to take anti-depressants (after a reasoned discussion).

Use the SPC as a guide to dose of gabapentin according to the patient's level of renal function.

See: www.medicines.org.uk/EMC/medicine/17095/SPC

Warn the patient about dizziness and somnolence, and explain that – if they can tolerate them – they should settle after the dose has been stable for three weeks. The tablets need to be taken regularly and can take four to six weeks to have their full effect.

Drivers and people who operate heavy machinery should be advised to be cautious about the somnolence side effect. If it is significant, they will need to avoid these activities until it settles. It may be best to start the tablets at the weekend.

If treatment is ineffective or the patient has surgical decompression of the nerve and no longer needs gabapentin, they should withdraw from treatment slowly, over not less than a week. (Sudden withdrawal can cause anxiety, insomnia, nausea, pain and sweating.) We suggest reducing the dose by 100–300mg every three days.

4.4 Pregabalin

Licensed for neuropathic pain. Pregabalin is cost effective in the neuropathic pain setting, hence its recommendation as a first-line treatment for non-diabetic neuropathic pain in the NICE 2010 guidance. It is also recommended as a second-line treatment by NICE for painful diabetic neuropathy. It does not require the lengthy titration of gabapentin, is tolerated well and benefits can be seen at one week.

Mechanism of action

Like gabapentin, pregabalin binds to the alpha2-delta subunit of the voltage-dependent calcium ion channel in the central nervous system, blocking channel action and thus calcium influx. However, the exact mechanism of action is unknown.

Evidence grading

Grade A evidence for chronic neuropathic pain and fibromyalgia (Moore *et al.* 2009).

NICE guidance weblink

Neuropathic pain: http://guidance.nice.org.uk/CG96

Preparations

- Capsules (25mg, 50mg, 75mg, 100mg, 150mg, 200mg, 225mg, 300mg)

Dosage

75–300mg twice daily

SPC weblink

www.medicines.org.uk/EMC/medicine/14651/SPC

Side effects

Dizziness, drowsiness, visual disturbance, ataxia, dysarthria, euphoria, oedema, tremor, lethargy, memory impairment, weight gain, constipation, dry mouth.

Caution

Renal impairment dose needs to be reduced. Check SPC for suggestions on dose according to renal function. Elderly patients may be prone to falls with dizziness. **See: www.medicines.org.uk/EMC/medicine/14651/SPC**

Contra-indications

Hypersensitivity to pregabalin. Pregnancy and breast-feeding.

Interactions

- Other central nervous system depressants, including sedatives, phenothiazines, and alcohol, may result in sedation.

Prescribing advice

Use the twice-daily dosage (which is cheaper than three times a day dosage and effective in the pain trials). Start at 75mg daily and increase after a week to 75mg twice a day. This dose is usually effective but it can be increased to 300mg twice a day if necessary. The main side effect is somnolence. Warn the patient of this and see if they can tolerate it initially, as it may settle after a few weeks. In the elderly, side-effect-prone individuals and patients with renal impairment, start with the 25mg dosage. Treatment should be withdrawn slowly because sudden withdrawal can cause anxiety, insomnia, nausea, pain and sweating. Stop treatment gradually, over one week.

4.5 Duloxetine hydrochloride

Duloxetine hydrochloride is licensed to treat pain related to diabetic peripheral neuropathy. It is a first-line treatment recommendation in 'NICE neuropathic pain guidance 2010'.

Mechanism of action

Duloxetine is a reuptake inhibitor of serotonin and noradrenaline, which lacks affinity for monoamine receptors within the central nervous system.

Evidence grading

Grade A evidence for diabetic peripheral neuropathy, fibromyalgia and osteoarthritis (OA) of the knee (Häuser *et al.* 2013; Hochberg *et al.* 2012; Lunn, Hughes & Wiffen 2009).

NICE guidance weblink

Neuropathic pain: http://guidance.nice.org.uk/CG96

Preparation

- Capsules (30mg, 60mg)

Dosage

60mg once daily and twice daily

SPC weblink

http://www.medicines.org.uk/EMC/medicine/15694/SPC

Side effects

Most commonly (in more than 10% of patients): headache, somnolence, nausea, dry mouth, diarrhoea, anxiety, decreased libido, agitation, abnormal dreams, dizziness, tremor, nervousness, paraesthesia, blurred vision, palpitations, yawning, constipation, vomiting, dyspepsia, flatulence, increased sweating, rash, musculoskeletal pain, muscle tightness, erectile dysfunction, fatigue, abdominal pain, decreased appetite.

Withdrawal symptoms when treatment is discontinued are common. These include dizziness, sensory disturbances, sleep disturbances, agitation or anxiety, nausea and vomiting, tremor, and headache.

Cautions

A history of mania or seizures, increased intra-ocular pressure or those at risk of acute narrow-angle glaucoma, pre-existing hypertension. Medical conditions which could be compromised by tachycardia or hypertension. Those at increased risk for hyponatraemia, such as the elderly, patients with cirrhosis or dehydration, or patients treated with diuretics.

Contra-indications

Hypersensitivity or intolerance to duloxetine, liver disease resulting in hepatic impairment, severe renal impairment (creatinine clearance <30ml/min), uncontrolled hypertension. Pregnancy and breast-feeding.

Interactions

- Other central nervous system depressants, including sedatives, phenothiazines and alcohol, may result in sedation.
- Monoamine oxidase inhibitors (MAOIs) or, within three weeks of such therapy, enhanced sedative effect of opioid or anti-depressant effect of MAOI. SSRIs, tricyclic anti-depressants, St John's Wort, venlafaxine, or triptans, tramadol, pethidine and tryptophan may increase risk of serotonin syndrome development
- Drugs that are predominantly metabolised by CYP2D6 (e.g. risperidone, tricyclic anti-depressants, particularly if they have a narrow therapeutic index such as flecainide, propafenone, and metoprolol).
- Anticoagulants and antiplatelet agents – potential increased risk of bleeding and increases in INR values have been reported when duloxetine has been co-prescribed with warfarin.
- Potent inhibitors of CYP1A2, like fluvoxamine, inhibit metabolism of duloxetine and should not be used together.
- Inducers of CYP1A2: smokers have almost 50% lower plasma concentrations of duloxetine compared with non-smokers.

Prescribing advice

For diabetic peripheral neuropathy pain, the starting dose of duloxetine is 60mg per day, which can be increased to 60mg twice daily. Duloxetine has been shown to treat pain symptoms in patients with fibromyalgia at a dose of 60mg twice daily (Arnold *et al.* 2005; Lunn, Hughes & Wiffen 2009). However, this is 'off label' (unlicensed indication) prescribing.

In patients with fibromyalgia who are sensitive to the side effects of medication, we suggest starting at 30mg once a day, increasing on a fortnightly basis to 60mg twice a day or highest tolerated dose.

Because of the withdrawal side effects of duloxetine, it should be gradually tapered when discontinuing treatment over a period of not less than two weeks, according to the patient's needs.

Monitoring

In patients with known hypertension or other cardiac disease, blood pressure monitoring is recommended, especially during the first month of treatment.

4.6 Capsaicin

Derived from chilli pepper plants and licensed for use in osteoarthritis (OA) and peripheral neuropathy, capsaicin is only mildly effective but may be suitable for patients who cannot tolerate or respond to other treatments. According to the NICE OA CG59 guidance, it should be considered for use in patients with hand and knee OA, alongside core OA treatment.

Mechanism of action

The chemical compound capsaicin (8-methyl-N-vanillyl-6-nonenamide), if used regularly, results in the neurotransmitter, substance P, being depleted from neurones.

Evidence grading

Grade A evidence for chronic pain and neuropathic pain (Derry *et al.* 2009; Kosuwon 2010; Mason *et al.* 2004a).

NICE guidance weblink

Osteoarthritis: http://guidance.nice.org.uk/CG59

Preparation

- Topical cream (0.025%, 0.075%)

Dosage

For osteoarthritis, 0.025% cream applied four times daily.

For painful diabetic peripheral neuropathy and herpes zoster neuralgic pain, 0.075% cream applied four times daily for eight weeks (then review).

SPC weblink

http://www.medicines.org.uk/EMC/medicine/269/SPC

Side effects

Initial burning sensations may be distressing but will reduce after the first few applications.

Caution

Avoid contact with eyes, and inflamed or delicate skin. Not to be used under tight bandages. Allergy to chillies.

Contra-indication

Hypersensitivity to any of the constituents.

Prescribing advice

Tell the patient to apply only a pea-size amount of cream to the affected area four times daily and not more often than every 4 hours. The cream should be rubbed in until there is no residue left on the skin surface. The applying finger should be washed immediately after application of the cream.

Advise the patient that the analgesic effect usually begins within the first week of treatment and increases with continuing regular application for the next two to eight weeks. Patients should avoid taking a shower or hot bath just before or after applying capsaicin, as it can increase the burning sensation.

For use of the 0.075% cream, hospital consultant supervision is currently recommended.

4.7 Lidocaine topical plasters

Lidocaine 5% topical medicated plasters are licensed for post-herpetic neuropathic pain. They are also recommended by NICE as a third-line treatment in painful peripheral neuropathy when use of oral medications is limited by co-morbidity or side effects.

Mechanism of action

A local analgesic effect is thought to be produced due to stabilisation of neuronal membranes and down-regulation of sodium channels.

Evidence grading

Grade A in neuropathic pain (Challapalli *et al.* 2005; Wolff *et al.* 2010).

NICE guidance weblink

Neuropathic pain: http://guidance.nice.org.uk/CG96

Preparation

- Topical medicated plaster (5%)

Dosage

One to three plasters for 12 hours, per 24 hours. Each 10cm x 14cm plaster contains 700 mg (5% w/w) lidocaine (50mg lidocaine per gram adhesive base).

SPC weblink

www.medicines.org.uk/emc/medicine/19291

Side effects

On the application site, some patients get erythema, rash or pruritis.

Caution

Avoid contact with eyes, mucous membranes, and inflamed, broken or delicate skin. The plasters should be used with caution in patients with severe cardiac impairment, severe renal impairment, severe hepatic impairment or those using Class I antiarrhythmic medicinal products (e.g. tocainide, mexiletine) and other local anaesthetics, since the risk of additive systemic effects cannot be excluded. Not recommended in pregnancy or lactation, as they have not been fully evaluated in humans in that situation.

One of the lidocaine metabolites, has been shown to be genotoxic and carcinogenic in rats. Secondary metabolites have been shown to be mutagenic. The clinical significance of this finding is unknown. Consequently, long-term treatment with the plasters is only justified if there is a therapeutic benefit for the patient.

Contra-indications

Hypersensitivity to any of the constituents or amide anaesthetics.

Prescribing advice

The painful area should be covered with the plaster (adjusted for size if necessary), or plasters, once a day for up to 12 hours within a 24-hour period. In total, not more than three plasters should be used at the same time.

Each plaster must be applied to the skin immediately after removal from the sachet and following removal of the release liner from the gel surface. Hairs in the affected area must be cut off with a pair of scissors (not shaved).

Response to treatment should be re-evaluated after two to four weeks. Treatment should be reassessed at regular intervals to decide whether the number of plasters needed to cover the painful area can be reduced, or if the plaster-free period can be extended.

Chapter 5

Non-steroidal anti-inflammatory drugs (NSAIDs)

5.1 Overview

NSAIDs are licensed for mild to moderate pain and inflammation in rheumatic disease and other musculoskeletal disorders. They have analgesic, antipyretic and anti-inflammatory effect and can be combined with other painkillers. This chapter will cover traditional NSAIDs (specifically ibuprofen, diclofenac and naproxen), Cox-2 NSAIDs (specifically celecoxib and etoricoxib) and topical NSAIDs.

Guidance on the use of NSAIDs is included in the osteoarthritis (OA), rheumatoid arthritis (RA), back pain and chronic kidney disease NICE guidance. If NSAIDs are to be prescribed long-term, it is cost effective to co-prescribe them with a generic proton pump inhibitor at lowest acquisition cost for all patients with OA and for those over the age of 45 years (NICE low back pain guidance 2009).

5.2 Traditional, non-selective and Cox 2 selective NSAIDs

Mechanism of action

NSAIDs work by cyclo-oxygenase inhibition of the prostaglandin pain pathway in the peripheral nervous system. With cyclo-oxygenase isoenzyme 2 inhibitors, they preferentially inhibit prostaglandins involved in pain and inflammation above cyclo-oxygenase 1 inhibitors that are involved in constitutional functions, such as gastroprotection.

Evidence grading

Grade A evidence in acute pain, chronic back pain, RA, OA, gout, ankylosing spondylitis (Moore *et al.* 2011a; Roelofs *et al.* 2008; Shi *et al.* 2004; Towheed *et al.* 2006; van den Berg *et al.* 2012; Zhang 2006).

NICE guidance weblinks

Osteoarthritis: http://guidance.nice.org.uk/CG59
Low back pain: http://guidance.nice.org.uk/CG88
Rheumatoid arthritis: http://guidance.nice.org.uk/CG79

Preparations

See Dosage.

Dosage – examples of traditional or non-selective NSAIDs

Ibuprofen:

1.2–1.8g per day in 3–4 divided doses; maximum dose 2.4g per day.
Available over the counter as:

- Tablets (200mg, 400mg)
- Oral suspension, syrup or granules
- Modified-release tablets (800mg) or capsules (300mg)

Naproxen:

For acute pain, 500mg initially (750mg in gout), followed by 250mg every 6–8 hours. For chronic rheumatic disease, 250–500mg twice a day.
Available as:

- Tablets (250mg, 375mg, 500mg)

Diclofenac:

150mg per day in 2–3 divided doses.
Available as:

- Tablets (25mg, 50mg)
- Modified-release capsules and tablets (75mg, 100mg)
- Suppositories (12.5 mg, 25mg, 50mg, 100mg)

Dosage – examples of Cox 2 selective NSAIDs

Celecoxib:

For OA and elderly patients, 200mg per day in 1–2 divided doses

For RA, 200–400mg/day in 2 divided doses.

Available as:

- Capsules (100mg and 200mg)

SPC weblink:

www.medicines.org.uk/EMC/medicine/14534/SPC

Etoricoxib:

For acute gout, 120mg daily for maximum of 7 days.

For OA, 30mg (starting dose for patients with OA) and 60mg per day tablet.

For RA, 90mg per day tablet.

SPC weblink:

www.medicines.org.uk/EMC/medicine/8734/SPC

Side effects

Nausea, vomiting, dyspepsia, abdominal pain, flatulence, diarrhoea, vomiting blood, malaena, peptic ulcers, perforation, fluid retention, worsens asthma, hypertension, rashes including photosensitivity. Nephrotoxicity in various forms, including interstitial nephritis, nephrotic syndrome and renal failure. Also abnormal liver function, hepatitis and jaundice. Visual disturbances, optic neuritis, headaches, paraesthesia, reports of aseptic meningitis, confusion, hallucinations, tinnitus, vertigo, dizziness, malaise, fatigue and drowsiness.

Cautions

- In elderly and patients with cardiovascular, renal and hepatic impairment, NSAIDs cause a dose-dependent reduction in prostaglandin formation and can precipitate renal failure. Renal function should be monitored in these patients.
- Patients with a history of heart failure and hypertension, since fluid retention and oedema have been reported in association with the use of NSAIDs.
- Cyclooxygenase 2 specific inhibitors and patients with risk factors for developing heart disease.
- Patients with asthma, since NSAIDs have been reported to cause bronchospasm.
- A history of gastrointestinal (GI) disease (such as ulcerative colitis or Crohn's disease), as these conditions may be exacerbated.

- Patients with systemic lupus erythematosus (SLE) and mixed connective tissue disorders. There may be an increased risk of aseptic meningitis.
- In women attempting to conceive, the use of NSAIDs may impair female fertility and is not recommended. In women who have difficulties conceiving or who are undergoing investigation of infertility, withdrawal of NSAIDs should be considered.
- For patients already having aspirin therapy, consider other analgesics first, as there is a high risk of GI complications (NICE OA guidance CG59).

Contra-indications

Patients with a known sensitivity to any of their constituents or in response to ibuprofen, aspirin, or other NSAIDs. Patients with a history of, or active, peptic ulcer, and patients with a history of, or active, upper GI bleeding or perforation related to previous NSAID therapy. Severe liver, renal or cardiac failure. During the last trimester of pregnancy. Combined with other NSAIDs, including the cyclooxygenase 2 specific inhibitors.

Etoricoxib is contra-indicated in patients with hypertension whose blood pressure is not under control.

Cyclooxygenase 2 specific inhibitors are contra-indicated in ischaemic heart disease, cerebrovascular disease, peripheral vascular disease and moderate or severe heart failure.

Interactions

- Lithium: may increase plasma concentrations and decrease elimination of lithium.
- Cardiac glycosides: increase plasma glycoside levels.
- Anticoagulants: may enhance the effects of anticoagulants, such as warfarin.
- Antidiabetic agents: isolated reports of hyperglycaemic and hypoglycaemic effects, which have required adjustments to the dosage of hypoglycaemic agents.
- Ciclosporin: nephrotoxicity may be increased by the effect of NSAIDs on renal prostaglandins.
- Mifepristone: NSAIDs should not be used for 8–12 days after mifepristone administration, as NSAIDs can reduce the effect of mifepristone.

- Quinolone antibiotics: patients taking NSAIDs and quinolones may have an increased risk of developing convulsions.
- Therapy with aspirin may increase the frequency of side effects.
- Corticosteroids can increase the risk of GI bleeding.
- Diuretics: inhibit the activity of diuretics. Diuretics can increase the risk of nephrotoxicity of NSAIDs. Concomitant treatment with potassium-sparing diuretics may be associated with increased serum potassium levels. Serum potassium should therefore be monitored.
- Anti-hypertensives: reduced anti-hypertensive effect.
- Tacrolimus: possible increased risk of nephrotoxicity when NSAIDS are given with tacrolimus.

Prescribing advice

When prescribing an NSAID, consider the risks of serious gastro-intestinal complication and cardiovascular disease. The cardiovascular risk associated with the prescribing of NSAIDs has been highly publicised and new guidance is produced at regular intervals. The British National Formulary has the latest Committee on Safety of Medicines (CSM) advice. Also be aware of NICE and European Medicines Agency (EMEA) guidance on NSAIDs.

The most recent advice has been that all NSAIDs (non-selective or selective COX 2 inhibitors) can increase blood pressure by 3–5mmHg, an amount that explains the increase in stroke, angina and heart failure seen in recent studies (Madhok *et al*. 2006; McGettigan & Henry 2011). We suggest that you try to avoid all NSAIDs in patients who have ischaemic heart and/or cerebrovascular disease.

The high risk groups for GI complications are: those aged over 65; patients concomitantly using medications that are likely to increase GI side effects (such as anticoagulants or corticosteroids); and those with serious co-morbidity, requiring prolonged use of maximum recommended doses of standard NSAIDs, with a previous history of peptic ulcer with or without complications. In these patients, if an NSAID is justified acutely then gastroprotection (lowest acquisition cost proton pump inhibitor) and NSAID will be required. However, the prescription of proton pump inhibitors does increase the risk of clostridium difficile infection, and proton pump inhibitor prescriptions should be regularly reviewed.

Try to use the lowest effective dose of NSAID for the shortest possible duration of treatment. Most are taken with food.

NSAIDs have a highly variable effect between patients so it is always worth trying two or three to find one that suits that individual, but allow up to four weeks of taking the NSAID on a regular basis for full anti-inflammatory effect.

To treat an acute attack of gout, use NSAIDs at their highest licensed dose and tailor down the dose as the signs of inflammation settle. Those NSAIDs that have been shown to be effective in gout are indometacin, piroxicam and etoricoxib (Cobra, Cobra & Cobra 1983; Schumacher, Jr. *et al.* 2002). With etoricoxib, the manufacturer advises that the patient's blood pressure should be checked three weeks after starting the drug.

5.3 Topical NSAIDs

Effective in the treatment of OA of superficial joints such as the knee, acute musculoskeletal injuries, periarthritis, epicondylitis, tendinitis, and tenosynovitis. Recommended in NICE OA guidance, for hand and knee OA, prior to considering opioids and oral NSAIDs.

Mechanism of action

Inhibits prostaglandin synthesis and release through inhibition of the cyclo-oxygenase enzyme.

Evidence grading

Grade A evidence for treatment of acute musculoskeletal conditions and chronic hand and knee OA (Derry, Moore & Rabbie 2012; Massey *et al.* 2010).

NICE guidance weblink

Osteoarthritis: http://guidance.nice.org.uk/CG59

Preparations

Available over the counter:

- Gels, cutaneous solution, foam, gel patch

Dosage

Apply to the affected area two to four times daily, except patch (apply one patch for 72 hours).

Side effects

Mild to moderate local irritation, erythema, pruritus and dermatitis and photosensitive skin reaction. Minor GI side effects such as nausea, dyspepsia, abdominal pain, and dyspnoea.

Caution

Patients with impaired liver or renal function.

Contra-indications

Hypersensitivity to constituents or in response to ibuprofen, aspirin or other NSAIDs.

Prescribing advice

Avoid eyes and mucosal surfaces. Do not apply to any sites affected by open skin lesions, skin diseases or infection. To avoid possibility of photosensitivity, advise patients against excessive exposure of treated area to sunlight. Effectiveness only demonstrated in short-term use. Review prescription after two to four weeks.

Chapter 6

Disease-modifying anti-rheumatic drugs (DMARDs)

6.1 Overview

Disease-modifying anti-rheumatic drugs (DMARDs) can suppress the inflammatory disease process and reduce the progression of disease. Be aware that this is a specialist area. NICE guidance on the management of rheumatoid arthritis (RA) has been provided and should be followed in conjunction with the British Society of Rheumatology/BSD/BHPR DMARD monitoring guidance. For patients with very active inflammatory disease Biologic therapy is available if the patients fulfil the NICE criteria for their use. Biologic therapy is initiated by Consultant Rheumatologists with expertise in the use of this therapy.

NICE (2008). Ankylosing spondylitis – adalimumab, etanercept and infliximab TA143:
http://guidance.nice.org.uk/TA143

NICE (2011). Ankylosing spondylitis – golimumab TA233:
http://guidance.nice.org.uk/TA233

NICE (2010). Psoriatic arthritis – etanercept, infliximab and adalimumab TA199:
http://guidance.nice.org.uk/TA199

NICE (2011). Psoriatic arthritis – golimumab TA220:
http://guidance.nice.org.uk/TA220

NICE (2007). Rheumatoid arthritis – adalimumab, etanercept and infliximab TA130:
http://guidance.nice.org.uk/TA130

NICE (2010). Rheumatoid arthritis – certolizumab pegol TA186:
http://guidance.nice.org.uk/TA186

NICE (2010). Rheumatoid arthritis – drugs for treatment after failure of a TNF inhibitor TA195:
http://guidance.nice.org.uk/TA195

NICE (2011). Rheumatoid arthritis (after the failure of previous anti-rheumatic drugs) – golimumab TA225:
http://guidance.nice.org.uk/TA225

NICE (2011). Rheumatoid arthritis (methotrexate-naïve) – golimumab (terminated appraisal) TA224:
http://guidance.nice.org.uk/TA224

NICE (2012). Rheumatoid arthritis – tocilizumab (rapid review TA198) TA247:
http://guidance.nice.org.uk/TA247

NICE (2013). Rheumatoid arthritis – abatacept (2nd line) (rapid review of TA234) TA280:
http://guidance.nice.org.uk/TA280

All consultations provide opportunities for education. Before commencing a new DMARD, we recommend a minimum of half an hour spent on patient education.

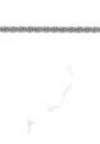

Table 6.1: Indications for DMARDs

	Rheumatoid arthritis	Psoriatic arthritis	SLE
Methotrexate	✔	✓	✓
Metoject® (subcutaneous methotrexate)	✔	✔	
Sulfasalazine	✔	✓	
Leflunomide	✔	✔	
Hydroxychloroquine	✔		✔

Denotes use ✓
Denotes licensed indication ✔

6.2 Methotrexate

Mechanism of action
Methotrexate inhibits the metabolism of rapidly dividing cells and is classed as an antimetabolite drug. Methotrexate reduces folic acid required for DNA synthesis by binding to the site of dihydrofolate reductase.

Evidence grading
Grade A evidence for rheumatoid arthritis (RA) and psoriatic arthritis. In RA, it is effective in controlling disease progression, including radiographic damage, and has a substantial clinical and statistically significant benefit (Jones, Crotty & Brooks 2000; Knevel *et al.* 2010; Suarez-Almazor *et al.* 1998a).

NICE guidance weblink
Rheumatoid arthritis: http://guidance.nice.org.uk/CG79

Preparations
- Tablets, subcutaneous injection, intramuscular injection

Dosage

Methotrexate may be given orally, or via intramuscular or subcutaneous routes.

The dose range for oral methotrexate is a minimum dose of 7.5mg weekly, usually with a maximum of 20mg weekly. Local protocols may agree a maximum of 30mg weekly.

The dose may be escalated by 2.5mg–5mg every two to four weeks, following review of disease activity, until remission is achieved or the maximum weekly dose has been reached. Remission may be defined as no synovitis and/or a disease activity score (DAS) of <2.6 (Luqmani *et al.* 2006). The DAS 28 is a validated tool to assess disease activity.

Be aware that only 2.5mg tablets should be prescribed and dispensed. This prevents the potential for accidental overdose/error when using low-dose methotrexate, as 10mg tablets can look identical to 2.5mg tablets. If acute methotrexate toxicity occurs, patients may require treatment with folinic acid.

Folic acid (5mg weekly) is given, to be taken on day three post-methotrexate and this may help to reduce the frequency of side effects.

If a patient is unable to tolerate oral methotrexate, or disease activity remains uncontrolled, consider using the subcutaneous (s/c) route. Refer to the Royal College of Nursing (RCN) guidance for teaching and administration of s/c methotrexate (www.rcn.org.uk).

Metoject® are methotrexate pre-filled syringes (intravenous, intramuscular, subcutaneous) 50mg/ml for the treatment of rheumatoid arthritis. These are available in ten weekly dosage forms: 7.5mg, 10mg, 12.5mg, 15mg, 17.5mg, 20mg, 22.5mg, 25mg, 27.5mg and 30mg.

SPC weblink

http://www.medicines.org.uk/EMC/medicine/22145/SPC

Side effects

Nausea, rash, mouth ulcers, diarrhoea, headache, hepatic toxicity, myelosuppression, mucositis, pancytopenia and rarely interstitial pneumonitis (this can be fatal in 15–20% of cases).

Cautions

Use with caution in the elderly. Use with extreme caution in patients with haematological depression, renal impairment, diarrhoea, and ulcerative disorders of the gastrointestinal (GI) tract or patients with a high alcohol intake.

Contra-indications

Hypersensitivity to any of the constituents. Significantly impaired renal or hepatic function. Pre-existing blood dyscrasias, such as significant marrow hypoplasia, leukopenia, thrombocytopenia or anaemia. Pregnancy and breast-feeding.

Interactions

- Trimethoprim: can precipitate aplastic anaemia.
- Penicillins and cephalosporins: increased toxicity of methotrexate (see Prescribing advice).
- Excretion of methotrexate probably reduced by NSAIDs, aspirin.
- Phenytoin has an additive anti-folate effect with methotrexate, and may also increase toxicity of methotrexate.
- Antimalarials increase anti-folate effect of methotrexate.
- Corticosteroids when given with methotrexate may increase risk of haematological toxicity.
- Probenecid: increased toxicity of methotrexate.
- Methotrexate may reduce absorption of digoxin.

Prescribing advice

Methotrexate is commonly the first-choice DMARD. However, the decision to commence methotrexate should take into account co-existing co-morbidity and patient preference. Consider the patient's social history such as whether or not they wish to start a family. Conception would not be advised, and adequate contraception is necessary prior to commencement of treatment. Excess alcohol (21 units for men and 14 units for women) should be avoided. Patients must be aware that, prior to conception, methotrexate should be discontinued for three months.

We suggest folic acid is given to help reduce the frequency of side effects of methotrexate. Many variations of the co-prescribing of folic acid with methotrexate exist across rheumatology departments. Usually, 5mg/day is given at least 24 hours after the methotrexate for one to three days. Folic acid should not be taken on the same day as methotrexate.

If prescribing trimethoprim, penicillins or cephalosporins (as no alternative), it is advisable to stop methotrexate for the duration of antibiotics. If a patient requires antibiotics and is systemically unwell, then methotrexate should be stopped for a minimum of one week. Live vaccines should be avoided (oral polio, MMR, yellow fever). Pneumococcal and annual influenza vaccines are recommended. Passive immunisation with varicella zoster immunoglobulin should be carried out in non-immune patients if exposed to chicken pox or shingles.

If a patient presents with acute shortness of breath whilst taking methotrexate (and up to four weeks after the last dose), this raises the suspicion of methotrexate pneumonitis and they should be assessed urgently by a rheumatology or respiratory specialist. If in doubt, stop the methotrexate. It is very important to warn the patient to report the development of respiratory symptoms whilst they are taking methotrexate. This should be stressed during the education session prior to commencing methotrexate.

Pre-treatment assessment

A pre-treatment assessment should be carried out (Chakravarty *et al.* 2008).

This should include full blood count (FBC), urea and electrolytes (U&E), liver function test (LFT) and chest x-ray (CXR) unless a CXR has been done within the last six months. Pulmonary function tests should be considered in selected patients.

Monitoring

The patient should be monitored (Chakravarty *et al.* 2008).

FBC, U&E, LFT should be carried out every two weeks until dose of methotrexate and monitoring stable for a period of six weeks; monthly thereafter until the dose and disease are stable for a year.

Thereafter monitoring may be reduced in frequency, based on clinical judgement with due consideration of risk factors (including age, co-morbidity and renal impairment) that would necessitate continued monthly monitoring.

6.3 Sulfasalazine

Sulfasalazine is licensed for the treatment of rheumatoid arthritis (RA). However, the onset of effect can be slow and a marked effect may not be seen for 6 to 12 weeks.

Mechanism of action

Sulfasalazine is a combination of 5-amino salicylic acid (anti-inflammatory effect) and sulfapyridine (carrier molecules). The exact mechanism of action is unknown.

Evidence grading

Grade A evidence for RA and psoriatic arthritis. In RA, it appears to have a clinically and statistically significant benefit on the disease activity. However, its effects on overall health status and radiological progression would appear to be modest (Suarez-Almazor *et al.* 1998b; Jones, Crotty & Brooks 2000). Several studies have indicated that sulfasalazine is effective in relieving the symptoms and slowing the progression of RA. Although it may show some effects within a month, it typically takes several months to be effective.

The decision to commence a DMARD such as sulfasalazine should be made taking into account co-existing co-morbidity and patient preference.

Preparations

- Enteric-coated tablets (500mg)
- Oral suspension (250mg/5ml)

Dosage

The dose is initially 500mg daily, increasing to 1g twice a day, over a four-week period.

Side effects

Nausea, rash, gastrointestinal (GI) intolerance, bruising. Harmless side effects such as urine stained orange. Some side effects may be dose-dependent and symptoms can sometimes be alleviated by reducing the dose.

Relative cautions

Pre-existing blood dyscrasias, such as significant marrow hypoplasia, leukopenia, thrombocytopenia or anaemia.

Contra-indications

Where there is a significant hypersensitivity to sulfasalazine, sulfonamides or salicylates.

Interactions

- Possibility that the uptake of digoxin and folate may be reduced.

Prescribing advice

Patients should be warned that it is not uncommon to develop an orange discoloration of their urine, and occasionally of their skin. This is a harmless side effect and should not cause alarm. The discoloration is temporary and disappears after stopping the medication. If a patient wears soft contact lenses, they may become stained. Sulfasalazine treatment is generally considered to be safe to use during pregnancy. However, it may cause reversible azoospermia in men.

Pre-treatment assessment

A pre-treatment assessment should be carried out (Chakravarty *et al.* 2008). Check FBC, U&E and LFTs.

Monitoring

The patient should be monitored (Chakravarty *et al.* 2008).

FBC and LFTs monthly for the first three months and three-monthly thereafter.

If, following the first year, dose and blood results remain stable, the frequency of blood tests can be reduced to every six months for the second year of treatment. Thereafter, monitoring may be discontinued.

The patient should be asked whether they have a rash or mouth ulcers at each visit.

6.4 Leflunomide

Leflunomide is licensed for the treatment of rheumatoid and psoriatic arthritis. Failure to tolerate methotrexate or sulfasalazine, and/or relevant co-existing co-morbidity and patient preference, would provide an indication for use. Consider the patient's social history such as whether or not they wish to start a family. As in the case of methotrexate, conception would not be advised and adequate contraception is necessary prior to commencement of treatment. If leflunomide is used in women of childbearing age, who wish to conceive later, contact the drug manufacturer for advice and support and they will advise on the required drug washout and blood-testing procedures.

Be aware that leflunomide has a lengthy half-life. In the event of a serious side effect, stop leflunomide and consider washout therapy. Colestyramine is usually suggested. We suggest 8g of colestyramine three times a day, for 11 days, for a full washout.

Blood pressure must be checked before commencing leflunomide treatment.

Mechanism of action

The active metabolite of leflunomide inhibits the human enzyme dihydroorotate dehydrogenase (DHODH) and exhibits anti-proliferative activity.

Evidence grading

Grade A evidence for rheumatoid arthritis (RA). Leflunomide appears to improve all clinical outcomes and delay radiographic progression at both 6 and 12 months of treatment, compared to placebo. Its efficacy and adverse events at two years of treatment are comparable to sulfasalazine and methotrexate. Long-term efficacy and toxicity remain to be established (Osiri *et al.* 2003; Golicki *et al.* 2012).

Preparations

- Tablets (10mg, 20mg, 100mg)

SPC weblink

www.medicines.org.uk/EMC/medicine/7480/SPC

Dosage

The maintenance dose for rheumatoid arthritis and psoriatic arthritis is 10mg–20mg once daily, depending on the severity (activity) of the disease.

Previously, a loading dose of 100mg daily, for three days, was given. Due to severe side effects related to this dosage, we are not aware the loading dose is still used.

Side effects

Nausea, diarrhoea, rash, pruritis, headache, GI intolerance, abdominal pain, alopecia and hypertension.

Cautions

Patients with impairment of liver function or moderate to severe renal insufficiency, impaired bone marrow function or significant anaemia, leucopenia, neutropenia or thrombocytopenia. History of tuberculosis.

Contra-indications

Severe immunodeficiency disorder (i.e. AIDS), severe infection, severe hypoproteinaemia (for example, in nephrotic syndrome). Pregnancy and breast-feeding. Hypersensitivity to any of the tablet constituents.

Interactions

- Leflunomide may enhance the anticoagulant effect of warfarin.
- Leflunomide may enhance the hypoglycaemic effect of tolbutamide.
- Leflunomide may increase the plasma concentration of phenytoin.

Prescribing advice

Start with 20mg dose, and reduce to 10mg if significant side effects develop. Due to severe side effects and increased risk of drug-induced pneumonitis associated with use of the loading dose (Chikura *et al.* 2009), the loading dose regime is rarely used.

Live vaccines should be avoided (i.e. oral polio, MMR and yellow fever). Pneumococcal and annual influenza vaccines are recommended. Excess alcohol should be avoided. The recommended weekly limits are 21 units for men and 14 units for women.

Passive immunisation with varicella zoster immunoglobulin should be carried out in non-immune patients if exposed to chicken pox or shingles.

Contraception should be maintained for at least two years for women and three months for men after treatment is discontinued or alternatively consider washout. Recommended washout is colestyramine (8g), administered three times a day, usually for 11 days. Alternatively, 50g of activated powdered charcoal may be administered four times a day.

Pre-treatment assessment

A pre-treatment assessment should be carried out (Chakravarty *et al.* 2008).

Check FBC and LFTs.

Check blood pressure. If >140/90mmHg on two consecutive readings two weeks apart, treat hypertension before commencing leflunomide.

Check weight – to allow assessment of weight loss that may be attributable to leflunomide.

Monitoring

The patient should be monitored (Chakravarty *et al.* 2008).

Check FBC and LFTs every month for six months and, if stable, two-monthly thereafter.

Continue to monitor FBC and LFTs monthly in the long term if co-prescribed with another immunosuppressant or potentially hepatotoxic agent.

Blood pressure and weight should be checked at each monitoring visit.

6.5 Hydroxychloroquine

Hydroxychloroquine is an anti-malarial. Hydroxychloroquine can help relieve the symptoms and slow down the progression of rheumatoid arthritis (RA). It is indicated for use in RA, juvenile chronic arthritis, discoid and systemic lupus erythematosus (SLE). Symptoms of RA should improve within six months.

Mechanism of action

Unknown.

Evidence grading

Grade A evidence for the treatment of RA (Gaujoux-Viala 2010; Suarez-Almazor *et al.* 2000). Its overall effect appears to be moderate, with a low toxicity profile. Its use in combination with other therapies is gaining acceptance (O'Dell *et al.*

2002). It is used widely in systemic lupus erythematosus (SLE), and Grade A evidence is available for its use during pregnancy in patients with SLE (Levy *et al.* 2001; Williams *et al.* 1994).

Preparations

- Tablets (200mg)

Dosage

Initially 400mg daily in divided doses, with a maintenance dose of 200–400mg daily. Treatment should be discontinued if there is no improvement in RA by six months. Be aware of any local protocols for the use of hydroxychloroquine.

Side effects

Nausea, diarrhoea, headache, rash, rarely visual changes or loss of vision, gastrointestinal (GI) symptoms. Very rarely, cardiac and generalised myopathy have been reported.

Cautions

Hepatic and renal impairment. Neurological disorders, severe GI disorders or porphyria. May exacerbate psoriasis and aggravate myasthenia gravis.

Contra-indications

Known hypersensitivity, pre-existing maculopathy of the eye.

Interactions

- Hydroxychloroquine has been reported to increase plasma digoxin levels.
- Absorption of hydroxychloroquine reduced by antacids.
- Amiodarone-increased risk of ventricular arrhythmias.

Prescribing advice

Enquire about any visual problems and suggest yearly visits to the optician.

Pre-treatment assessment

A pre-treatment assessment should be carried out (Chakravarty *et al.* 2008).

Check FBC, U&E, LFTs.

Ask about visual impairment (which is not corrected by glasses). Record near visual acuity of each eye (with reading glasses if worn), using a reading chart. If no abnormality detected, commence treatment. If abnormality detected, refer to optometrist.

Monitoring

The patient should be monitored (Chakravarty *et al.* 2008).

The Royal College of Ophthalmologists recommends an annual review either by an optometrist or the practitioner enquiring about visual symptoms, rechecking visual acuity and assessing for blurred vision, using the reading chart.

Patients should be advised to report any visual disturbance.

No blood monitoring is required.

Chapter 7

Osteoporosis and Paget's disease

7.1 Osteoporosis

Patients who have had a fragility fracture, or are at risk of osteoporosis from any other cause should be assessed and treated according to the current NICE osteoporosis guidance. The National Osteoporosis Guideline Group (www.shef.ac.uk/NOGG/) gives an overall risk assessment profile and guidance on treatment initiation for patients, which includes those patients taking corticosteroids.

Guidance on deciding whether DEXA scanning should be considered, for people at risk of osteoporosis, has been incorporated in the recent NICE guidance on assessing patients for osteoporosis.

See: www.nice.org.uk/CG146

Bisphosphonates are the first-line drug choices for osteoporosis treatment; denosumab, strontium ranelate, raloxifene, teriparatide and calcium and vitamin D supplementation will also be covered. HRT is not licensed for use as a treatment for osteoporosis and therefore will not be covered.

Table 7.1: Licensed dosages for osteoporosis treatments

	Prevention of post-menopausal osteoporosis	Treatment of post-menopausal osteoporosis	Treatment of osteoporosis in men	Treatment of corticosteroid-induced osteoporosis
Alendronic acid	10mg/day	10mg/day 70mg/week	10mg/day	10mg/day (women only)
Ibandronic acid		150mg/month IV 3mg every 3months		
Risedronate sodium	5mg/day	5mg/day 35mg/week	35mg/week	5mg/day (women only)
Zoledronic acid		IV 5mg/year	IV 5mg/year	IV 5mg/year
Denosumab	s/c 60mg every 6 months	s/c 60mg every 6 months		
Strontium	2g daily	2g daily		
Raloxifene	60mg daily	60mg daily		
Teriparatide		s/c 20 micrograms daily for 2 years	s/c 20 micrograms daily for 2 years	s/c 20 micrograms daily for 2 years

7.2 Paget's disease

A chronic bone disorder with disorganised bone growth, which can result in bone enlargement and deformity. The pain arising from this condition is usually unresponsive to standard analgesics and NSAIDs. The mainstay of treatment is with bisphosphonates; four have been used to treat Paget's disease (alendronate, etidronate, intravenous (IV) pamidronate and IV zoledronic acid). A higher dosage of bisphosphonate is generally used for Paget's disease than for osteoporosis. Oral risedronate and IV zoledronic acid are now licensed for this indication and most commonly used.

7.3 Bisphosphonates

General prescribing advice

Bisphosphonates are very poorly absorbed from the gastrointestinal (GI) tract. Correct dosing and administration of these preparations is key to achieving their effect. For evidence grading, preparations, dosage, cautions and contra-indications, see the individual drugs below.

- **A bisphosphonate is best taken immediately after getting up in the morning, on an empty stomach.**
- **Patients should be advised to take alendronic acid, ibandronic acid or risedronate sodium with a full glass of tap water and should not lie down for at least 30 minutes after taking their tablet.**
- **Use of these preparations may be ineffective due to non-compliance with the correct regime. In apparent non-responders, check that patients are taking the medicine correctly.**
- **Food and other drugs should not be taken for 1 hour after taking the tablet.**
- **Use with caution in 3B chronic kidney disease (CKD) renal impairment (see the individual drugs), and avoid in CKD 4 and 5.**
- **If calcium is required on the same day, this should be taken with a main meal later in the day.**
- **Wherever possible, advise the patient that all invasive dental work should be completed prior to commencement of bisphosphonate – because of the potential risk of avascular necrosis of the jaw. Good oral hygiene needs to be maintained throughout treatment.**

Mechanism of action

All the bisphosphonates prevent the breakdown of bone by osteoclasts.

Drug interactions

Other than the potential for interference with absorption (most notably with some foods, calcium and iron), there are no known drug interactions.

General cautions

Atypical femoral fractures have been reported with all bisphosphonates – see MHRA warning:

www.mhra.gov.uk/Safetyinformation/DrugSafetyUpdate/CON120213

If patients receiving this treatment develop hip, groin or thigh pain, arrange for bilateral femoral x-rays to look for this rare complication. Patients should be warned to report this symptom and the bisphosphonate should be stopped until assessment has been completed.

In 2013, the National Osteoporosis Society suggested that, after five years of oral bisphosphonates and three years of intravenous zoledronic acid therapy, risk benefit should be reassessed. With prolonged use of these medications, 'drug holidays' should be considered.

See: http://www.shef.ac.uk/NOGG/NOGG_Executive_Summary.pdf

Alendronic acid

NICE recommends alendronic acid as a first-line treatment for primary and secondary prevention of osteoporosis (2011 NICE guidance). All doses are licensed for use in post-menopausal women. Only 5mg/day and 10mg/day have a licence for male use. Only the 5mg/day dose is licensed for pre-menopausal women.

Evidence grading

Grade A evidence in fracture reduction vertebral and non-vertebral sites (Wells *et al.* 2008a).

NICE guidance weblinks

Primary prevention of osteoporosis: http://guidance.nice.org.uk/TA160

Secondary prevention of osteoporosis: http://guidance.nice.org.uk/TA161

Preparations

- Tablets (5mg, 10mg, 70mg)

Dosage

Treatment of post-menopausal women is 10mg daily or 70mg once per week.

Treatment of osteoporosis in men is 10mg per day.

Prevention of post-menopausal osteoporosis (in women not on HRT) 10mg per day.

Side effects

Oesophagitis, dysphagia, abdominal pain and distension, diarrhoea or constipation, flatulence, musculoskeletal pain, headache, rash, erythema, photosensitivity, uveitis, transient decrease in serum phosphate, nausea, vomiting. Peptic ulceration and hypersensitivity reactions also reported. Osteonecrosis of the jaw.

Cautions

Upper gastrointestinal (GI) disorders (such as dysphagia, symptomatic oesophageal disease, gastritis, duodenitis or ulcers). History (within one year) of ulcers, active GI bleeding or surgery of the upper GI tract, renal impairment (avoid if eGFR <35ml/min). Correct disturbances of calcium and mineral metabolism (such as vitamin D deficiency and hypocalcaemia) before starting bisphosphonates.

Contra-indications

Abnormalities of the oesophagus and other factors which delay emptying (for example, stricture or achalasia), hypocalcaemia, pregnancy or breast-feeding. Hypersensitivity to any of the tablet constituents.

Prescribing advice

Alendronic acid should be given with 'adequate calcium and vitamin D ingestion' and in most instances calcium supplements would be required. Trials used 500mg of calcium supplements and 250IU of vitamin D per day.

Patients should be advised to stop taking the tablets and refer to the doctor if they develop symptoms of oesophageal irritation such as dysphagia, new or worsening heartburn, pain on swallowing, or retrosternal pain.

Alendronic acid is also available as a 70mg tablet, which is taken once a week, on the same day each week.

Risedronate sodium

The recommended dose in Paget's disease is one 30mg tablet orally for 2 months. If re-treatment is considered necessary (at least 2 months post-treatment), a new treatment with the same dose and duration of therapy could be given.

Licensed for treatment of post-menopausal osteoporosis to reduce risk of hip or vertebral fracture (5mg/day and 35mg/week dose), prevention of corticosteroid-induced osteoporosis, and prevention of osteoporosis in post-menopausal women (5mg/day dose). Alternative first-line treatment, as recommended by NICE in 2011 osteoporosis guidance, if patients are unable to comply with alendronate oral regime or if they have contra-indications or side effects with alendronate, and T scores, independent risk factors and age fulfil their criteria for treatment according to NICE guidance.

Evidence grading

Grade A evidence in fracture reduction, vertebral and non-vertebral sites (Wells *et al.* 2002). Grade A evidence in Paget's disease of the bone (Miller *et al.* 1999).

NICE guidance weblinks

Primary prevention of osteoporosis: http://guidance.nice.org.uk/TA160
Secondary prevention of osteoporosis: http://guidance.nice.org.uk/TA161

Preparations

- Tablets (5mg, 30mg, 35mg)

Dosage

Treatment or prevention of osteoporosis (including corticosteroid-induced) in post-menopausal women: 5mg daily. Treatment of post-menopausal osteoporosis: 35mg once per week.

Paget's disease of the bone: 30mg daily for two months.

Side effects

Upper gastrointestinal (GI) symptoms – dyspepsia, nausea, diarrhoea, constipation, oesophageal stricture, and duodenitis; headache, musculoskeletal pain.

Cautions

Oesophageal abnormalities and other factors that delay transit or emptying (such as stricture and achalasia). Renal impairment – avoid if estimated glomerular filtration rate (eGFR) is <30ml/min. Correct disturbances of calcium and mineral metabolism before starting bisphosphonates.

Contra-indications

Hypocalcaemia, pregnancy and breast-feeding.

Prescribing advice

Reinforce the importance of taking bisphosphonates correctly or they will be ineffective.

Ibandronic acid

Ibandronic acid may be taken daily, but it is the only oral bisphosphonate that is approved to be taken monthly. Ibandronic acid is licensed to prevent and to treat osteoporosis in post-menopausal women.

Evidence grading

Grade A evidence for reduction of vertebral fractures with daily preparation (Harris *et al.* 2008; Bianchi *et al.* 2012).

Preparations

- Tablets (150mg)
- Intravenous injection (3mg/3ml)

Dosage

Licensed for treatment of post-menopausal osteoporosis. The dose of ibandronic acid is 150mg once-monthly. The dose of ibandronic acid intravenously is 3mg every three months.

Side effects

Flu-like symptoms (monthly preparation), musculoskeletal pain, dyspepsia, abdominal pain and diarrhoea.

Cautions

Renal impairment.

Contra-indications

Estimated glomerular filtration rate (eGFR) <30ml/min, hypocalcaemia, pregnancy and breast-feeding. Hypersensitivity to any of the tablet constituents.

Prescribing advice

If monthly dosing is used, the tablet should be taken on the same day of each month. Tablets should be taken at least 60 minutes before the first food or drink of the day (other than plain water) or before other oral medication, because of concern that food or medication will interfere with the absorption of ibandronic acid. Tablets should not be chewed or sucked, as this can cause irritation of the mouth and throat.

Zoledronic acid

The recommended dose in Paget's disease is one 5mg IV infusion. If re-treatment is considered necessary, it should be at least 1 year after the last treatment.

Zoledronic acid is a yearly intravenous bisphosphonate, licensed to treat osteoporosis in post-menopausal women, men and corticosteroid-induced osteoporosis.

Evidence grading

Grade A evidence for reduction of vertebral, non-vertebral and hip fractures. Reduced mortality post hip fracture also demonstrated (Jansen *et al*. 2012). Grade A evidence in Paget's disease (Reid *et al*. 2005).

Preparations

- Intravenous injection (5mg in 100ml solution)

SPC weblink

www.medicines.org.uk/EMC/medicine/18171/SPC

Dosage

For osteoporosis, the dose of zoledronic acid is 5mg every 12 months. For Paget's disease, the dose of zoledronic acid is 5mg as a single infusion.

Side effects

Flu-like symptoms, musculoskeletal pain, dyspepsia, abdominal pain and diarrhoea, avascular necrosis of jaw, atrial fibrillation.

Cautions

Renal impairment.

Contra-indications

Estimated glomerular filtration rate (eGFR) <35ml/min, hypocalcaemia, pregnancy and breast-feeding. Hypersensitivity to any of the constituents.

Prescribing advice

Advise the patient that all dental work should be completed prior to commencement of treatment. Plenty of fluids during day of infusion. Paracetamol recommended for flu-like symptoms, which should reduce with each infusion. Check calcium and renal function prior to infusion and correct if necessary. Re-enforce the importance of taking calcium and vitamin D supplements in addition to having the infusions.

7.4 Denosumab

Mechanism of action

A fully human monoclonal antibody. It is an antireceptor activator of nuclear factor Kappa B Ligand. Osteoclast function is inhibited, so preventing bone resorption.

Evidence grading

Grade A evidence for reduction of vertebral, non-vertebral and hip fractures (von Keyserlingk *et al.* 2011; Papapoulos *et al.* 2012). Approved by NICE October 2010 in secondary and primary prevention of post-menopausal osteoporosis when bisphosphonates are contra-indicated, not tolerated or ineffective. In primary prevention, restrictions around severity of T scores and risk factors need to be considered.

NICE guidance weblink

www.NICE.org.uk/TA204

Preparation

- Subcutaneous injection (60mg)

SPC weblink

www.medicines.org.uk/EMC/medicine/23127/SPC

Dosage

For prevention and treatment of post-menopausal osteoporosis: 60mg every six months.

Side effects

Can include urinary tract infection, upper respiratory tract infection, sciatica, cataracts, constipation, rash, pain in extremity, avascular necrosis of the jaw. Skin infections (predominantly cellulitis in the lower leg). Atypical femoral fractures have recently been reported by the MHRA. If patients receiving this treatment develop hip, groin or thigh pain, arrange for bilateral femoral x-rays to look for this rare complication. Patients should be warned to report this symptom and the treatment should be stopped until assessment has been completed.

See: www.mhra.gov.uk/Safetyinformation/DrugSafetyUpdate/CON239411

Cautions

Hypocalcaemia (must be corrected before treatment)

Contra-indications

Hypocalcaemia, pregnancy and breast-feeding. Hypersensitivity to any of the constituents.

Prescribing advice

Cost-effectiveness analysis has shown denosumab to be more cost-effective than strontium treatment. It also has the advantage of parenteral delivery and can be used in patients with significant renal impairment if hypocalcaemia has been corrected.

In patients at risk of hypocalcaemia, monitoring of calcium levels is recommended. Calcium levels should be checked before each injection and the injection should not be administered until calcium levels are in the normal range. Deaths have been attributed to hypocalcaemia from denosumab therapy when it has been given at the higher dosage for metastases.

Advise the patient that all invasive dental work should be completed prior to commencement of treatment and good oral hygiene maintained throughout treatment. In trials, hospitalisation with cellulitis was more common, so advise patient to seek medical attention early if concerned about skin infection.

7.5 Strontium ranelate

Licensed for the treatment of post-menopausal osteoporosis to reduce the risk of vertebral and hip fractures. Second-line treatment for primary prevention and secondary treatment of post-menopausal osteoporosis in NICE 2011 osteoporosis guidance after bisphosphonates if risk factors are severe enough.

Mechanism of action

Strontium ranelate is thought to have a dual effect on bone metabolism, increasing bone formation and decreasing bone resorption.

Evidence grading

Grade A evidence for vertebral and non-vertebral fracture reduction, grade B for hip fracture reduction (O'Donnell *et al.* 2006; Reginster *et al.* 2012; Ringe & Doherty 2010; Stevenson *et al.* 2007).

NICE guidance weblinks

Primary prevention of osteoporosis http://guidance.nice.org.uk/TA160
Secondary prevention of osteoporosis http://guidance.nice.org.uk/TA161

Preparation

- Sachet (2g)

SPC weblink

www.medicines.org.uk/EMC/medicine/15410/SPC

Dosage

The recommended dose is a 2g sachet once daily, taken as a suspension in water, 2 hours before eating.

Side effects

Nausea, diarrhoea, headache, dermatitis and creatinine kinase elevations. A serious adverse event associated with strontium ranelate therapy is an increased incidence of venous thromboembolism and pulmonary embolism. An MHRA safety update has necessitated a review of strontium ranelate's indications and contra-indications as an increased risk of serious cardiac disorders, including myocardial infarction, has been found. Life-threatening skin reactions (Stevens-Johnson syndrome (SJS), toxic epidermal necrolysis (TEN), and drug rash with eosinophilia and systemic symptoms (DRESS)) have been reported with the use of strontium.

Cautions

In patients at increased risk of venous thromboembolism, or high risk of cardiovascular events,

see: www.mhra.gov.uk/Safetyinformation/DrugSafetyUpdate/CON266148

Contra-indications

Severe renal impairment (creatinine clearance <30ml/min), hypersensitivity, pregnancy and breast-feeding.

Ischaemic heart disease, peripheral vascular disease, cerebrovascular disease, uncontrolled hypertension.

See: www.mhra.gov.uk/Safetyinformation/DrugSafetyUpdate/CON266148

Interactions

May prevent absorption of oral tetracycline or quinolone antibiotics.

Prescribing advice

This is an alternative treatment option for women for whom bisphosphonates are contra-indicated, or who are unable to comply with the special recommendations for use of bisphosphonates, or who cannot take them because of intolerance. Absorption of strontium ranelate is reduced by food, milk and dairy products. It should therefore be administered between meals, ideally at bedtime and preferably at least 2 hours before and after eating. Patients should be warned about the signs and symptoms and monitored closely for skin reactions. The highest risk of SJS or TEN is within the first weeks of treatment and usually around 3-6 weeks for DRESS. If symptoms or signs of SJS, TEN or DRESS occur, strontium treatment should be discontinued immediately.

7.6 Teriparatide

Prescribe, according to NICE 2011 guidance, either as treatment for women over 55 years of age with further fracture despite bisphosphonate or intolerance to bisphosphonate and strontium, or the combination of extremely low bone mineral density or very low bone density with two or more fractures and other risk factors for osteoporosis.

Mechanism of action

Teriparatide is a synthetic version of human parathyroid hormone, which is produced by the parathyroid glands. This hormone is involved in the metabolism of calcium and phosphorus. Teriparatide mimics the effects of the natural human hormone and is used to increase bone formation by direct effects on osteoblasts, indirectly increasing the intestinal absorption of calcium, increasing the tubular re-absorption of calcium and excretion of phosphate by the kidney.

Evidence grading

Grade A evidence for vertebral and non-vertebral fracture reduction in post-menopausal women with previous fractures (Han & Wan 2012).

NICE guidance weblinks

Primary prevention of osteoporosis: http://guidance.nice.org.uk/TA160
Secondary prevention of osteoporosis: http://guidance.nice.org.uk/TA161

Preparation

- Injection (250micrograms/ml 3ml pre-filled pen intended for 28 doses)

SPC weblink

www.medicines.org.uk/EMC/medicine/12561/SPC

Dosage

20 micrograms daily for a maximum duration of 24 months (course not to be repeated)

Side effects

Pain, swelling, redness, bruising or itching around injection site, limb pain, nausea and vomiting, dizziness, headache, fatigue, depression, chest pain, muscle cramps, vertigo, dyspnoea, raised cholesterol levels, increased sweating, anaemia, asthenia, palpitations, sciatica, hypotension, gastro-oesophageal reflux, polyuria, weight gain.

Cautions

Moderate renal impairment, people who have (or have recently had) stones in the urinary tract.

Contra-indications

Severe renal impairment, metabolic bone diseases other than osteoporosis (such as Paget's disease of bone), hyperparathyroidism, hypercalcaemia, bone cancer, previous radiotherapy to the bones, unexplained raised levels of alkaline phosphatase, pregnancy, breast-feeding. Hypersensitivity to any of the constituents.

Interactions

- Digoxin, as teriparatide causes temporary increases in the blood level of calcium, and this may potentially predispose people to side effects associatedwith digoxin.

Prescribing advice

In short-term clinical studies with teriparatide, isolated episodes of transient postural hypotension were observed. Typically, an event began within 4 hours of dosing and spontaneously resolved within a few minutes to a few hours. When transient postural hypotension occurred, it happened within the first few doses, was relieved by lying down, and did not prevent continued treatment.

7.7 Raloxifene

Raloxifene is licensed for the prevention and treatment of osteoporosis in post-menopausal women. It is also recommended as a second-line treatment for secondary post-menopausal osteoporosis in the NICE 2011 osteoporosis guidance, after bisphosphonates, if the risk factors are severe enough. Raloxifene is not indicated for the treatment of menopausal symptoms.

Mechanism of action

Raloxifene is a selective oestrogen receptor modulator (SERM), which has an agonist effect on bone.

Evidence grading

Grade A evidence for vertebral and non-vertebral fracture reduction (Kanis *et al.* 2010) in post-menopausal women.

NICE guidance weblinks

Primary prevention of osteoporosis: http://guidance.nice.org.uk/TA160

Secondary prevention of osteoporosis: http://guidance.nice.org.uk/TA161

Preparations

- Tablets (60mg)

SPC weblink

www.medicines.org.uk/EMC/medicine/595/SPC

Dosage

Give 60mg once daily.

Side effects

Venous thrombo-embolism, thrombo-phlebitis. It should not be used within one year of the menopause because of an increased incidence of vasomotor symptoms. Other side effects include leg cramps, peripheral oedema, and flu-like symptoms.

Cautions

Risk factors for venous thrombo-embolism, active breast cancer (avoid use).

Contra-indications

History of venous thromboembolism, undiagnosed uterine bleeding, endometrial cancer, liver impairment, cholestasis, severe renal impairment, pregnancy and breast-feeding. Hypersensitivity to any of the tablet constituents.

Interactions

- Colestyramine (or other anion exchange resins), which significantly reduces the absorption and enterohepatic cycling of raloxifene.
- Anticoagulant effect of warfarin antagonised.

Prescribing advice

The 2011 NICE guidance on osteoporosis advises that this medication should not be used for primary prevention of osteoporosis, and in secondary treatment it should only be considered after bisphosphonates in patients with very low T scores or patients from older age groups. With the benefits of treatment from recently licensed intravenous zoledronic acid and subcutaneous denosumab, the use of raloxifene has greatly diminished. This preparation should only be given to women who have no menopausal symptoms, at least 12 months after their last period.

7.8 Calcium with or without vitamin D supplements

Licensed to be an adjunct to conventional therapy in the prevention and treatment of osteoporosis.

Mechanism of action

Supplement for when dietary intake of calcium is insufficient.

Evidence grading

Grade A evidence that calcium supplementation, with or without vitamin D, results in reduction in fracture rate (Avenell *et al.* 2009; Tang *et al.* 2012), particularly in patients with an inadequate dietary intake.

Preparations

- Tablets, effervescent tablets, chewable tablets, granules, powder and syrup (various strengths)

Dosage

Supplements should aim to achieve a total intake (including dietary sources) of 1200–1500mg elemental calcium per day. Usually 1–2 tablets.

Side effects

Constipation, flatulence, nausea, abdominal pain and diarrhoea – usually mild.

Cautions

Renal impairment, sarcoidosis, pregnancy and breast-feeding.

Contra-indications

Conditions associated with hypercalcaemia and hypercalciuria. Hypersensitivity to any of the tablet constituents.

Interactions

- Thiazide diuretics reduce the urinary excretion of calcium. Due to increased risk of hypercalcaemia, serum calcium should be regularly monitored during concomitant use of thiazide diuretics.
- Systemic corticosteroids reduce calcium absorption. During concomitant use, it may be necessary to increase the dose.
- Tetracycline preparations should be administered at least 2 hours before, or 4–6 hours after, oral intake of calcium.
- Hypercalcaemia may increase the toxicity of digoxin during treatment with calcium.
- If a bisphosphonate or sodium fluoride is used concomitantly, this preparation should be administered at least three hours before the intake of Calcichew D3 Forte® chewable tablets, since gastrointestinal absorption may be reduced.
- Oxalic acid (found in spinach and rhubarb) and phytic acid (found in whole cereals) may inhibit calcium absorption through formation of insoluble calcium salts. The patient should not take calcium products within two hours of eating foods high in oxalic acid and phytic acid.
- Absorption of levothyroxine, iron and zinc is reduced by calcium salts.

Prescribing advice

For patients who lack adequate exposure to the sun, (which includes most elderly patients for eight months of the year) or who have inadequate diet, or some degree of renal impairment, it may be necessary to provide vitamin D 400–800 IU daily (Fultium D3 is one example of a currently licensed vitamin D supplement). Elderly patients are at greatest risk and are likely to need Adcal-D3® or Calcichew D3 Forte® 2 tablets daily. Some of these patients with renal impairment will benefit from treatment with calcium (500mg daily) and 1 alpha calcidol (250 nanograms daily).

Monitoring

Ideally treatment should be monitored, by measuring plasma calcium levels.

Chapter 8

Gout

8.1 Overview

Gout is a common musculoskeletal condition caused by deposition of uric acid crystals in the joints (arthritis) or in the soft tissues (tophi). In an acute attack, the symptoms should be treated with non-steroidal anti-inflammatory drugs (NSAIDs), colchicine or corticosteroids, depending on the patient's co-morbidities. Once the acute attack has settled, a decision should be made about therapy to lower uric acid levels in the long term.

Both the licensed medications (allopurinol and febuxostat) are likely to precipitate acute flare-ups of gout during the first six months of therapy, and these treatments need to be taken continually through episodes once treatment has been agreed upon. For this reason, co-prescription of NSAIDs and colchicine is recommended. Once established on treatment, effective titration of the dose according to uric acid level is best practice to prevent flare-ups. Stopping the uric acid-lowering medications is likely to precipitate a flare-up of gout, so both prescriber and patient need to be certain that long-term therapy can be complied with.

8.2 Allopurinol

Allopurinol is used to prevent recurrent attacks of gout. It is not a treatment for acute gout.

Mechanism of action

Allopurinol is an isomer of hypoxanthine and inhibits the production of uric acid, the metabolite which causes gout, by inhibiting the enzyme xanthine oxidase. Allopurinol is rapidly metabolised to oxipurinol, which is also a xanthine oxidase inhibitor. NICE recommended this as the first-line therapy in treating hyperuricaemia in patients with gout, in their 2008 guidance.

Evidence grading

Grade A evidence for treatment of gout (Zhang *et al.* 2006).

NICE guidance weblink

http://guidance.nice.org.uk/TA164

Preparations

- Tablets (100mg, 300mg)

Dosage

100–600mg daily

Side effects

Rash, Stevens Johnson syndrome, hypersensitivity consisting of fever, eosinophilia and hepatitis, deterioration in renal function, nausea and vomiting, vertigo.

Cautions

Reduced doses should be used in patients with hepatic or renal impairment.

Contra-indications

Hypersensitivity to allopurinol, pregnancy, breast-feeding.

Interactions

- Azathioprine is metabolised to 6-mercaptopurine which is inactivated by the action of xanthine oxidase. Only 25% of the usual dose of 6-mercaptopurine or azathioprine should be given.
- Vidarabine (adenine arabinoside): the plasma half-life of vidarabine is increased in the presence of allopurinol.
- Chlorpropamide: increased risk of prolonged hypoglycaemic activity because allopurinol and chlorpropamide may compete for excretion in the renal tubule, particularly if renal function is poor.
- Increased effect of warfarin and other coumarin anticoagulants when co-administered with allopurinol.

- Theophylline: inhibition of the metabolism of theophylline may occur.
- Ampicillin/amoxicillin: an increase in incidence of skin rash can occur with concurrent use of allopurinol.
- Ciclosporin: plasma concentration of ciclosporin may be increased.
- Didanosine: a dose reduction of didanosine may be needed.

Prescribing advice

Start once the acute attack has settled or with NSAID/colchicine cover (500 micrograms twice daily). Serum urate level should respond after four weeks' treatment with allopurinol. Titrate the dose of allopurinol in 100mg increments monthly until uric acid is less than 0.36mmols/l (Zhang *et al*. 2006) or 0.3mmol/l (Jordan *et al*. 2007). It takes six months to see full effects, and gouty tophi reduction may take years. If gout is difficult to control, check the patient's adherence.

In patients without significant co-morbidity or renal impairment, start at 100mg and check plasma urate levels at four weeks. Increase in 100mg doses until urate is less than 0.36 mmol/l.

In patients with severe liver or renal impairment, start at 100mg per day and increase in 50mg increments. Monitor renal function as well as uric acid levels.

Allopurinol should be taken orally once a day after a meal. If the daily dosage exceeds 300mg and gastrointestinal side effects occur, dividing the dose may control the problem.

8.3 Febuxostat

Mechanism of action

Febuxostat is a 2-arylthiazole non-purine derivative that selectively inhibits xanthine oxidase. This reduces uric acid production, which is the metabolite that causes gout.

Evidence grading

Grade A evidence for treatment of gout (Schumacher *et al*. 2008; Tayar *et al*. 2012). Approved by NICE in 2008 as second-line therapy for gout if allopurinol is contra-indicated, or the patient is allopurinol-intolerant, or allopurinol has been titrated to maximum dosage and has not been effective.

NICE guidance weblink

http://guidance.nice.org.uk/TA164

Preparations

- Tablets (80mg, 120mg)

SP weblink

www.medicines.org.uk/EMC/medicine/22830/SPC

Dosage

80–120mg daily

Side effects

Rash, Stevens Johnson syndrome, nausea and vomiting, diarrhoea, abnormal liver function tests, headache.

Cautions

Patients with alteration of thyroid function: 5% of patients had elevation of TSH in studies on long-term use of febuxostat. Patients on theophylline.

Contra-indications

Hypersensitivity to febuxostat. Ischaemic heart disease, congestive cardiac failure, pregnancy and breast-feeding. Patients with hereditary problems of galactose intolerance, the Lapp lactase deficiency or glucose-galactose malabsorption should not take this medicine.

Interactions

- Azathioprine is metabolised to 6-mercaptopurine, which is inactivated by the action of xanthine oxidase. Only 25% of the usual dose of 6-mercaptopurine or azathioprine should be given.
- Theophylline: inhibition of the metabolism of theophylline may occur, leading to elevated levels of theophylline.

Prescribing advice

Check liver function tests (LFTs) before starting febuxostat. Start once the acute attack settled and with NSAID/colchicine cover (500 micrograms twice daily) at 80mg dose. The serum urate level should respond after 2–4 weeks' treatment with febuxostat. Increase to 120mg doses if urate is not less than 0.36 mmol/l.

As gout can flare up during the first six months of treatment, prophylaxis with NSAID or colchicine is recommended for six months. Periodically check LFTs as clinically indicated. It can take six months to see the full effects of treatment, and gouty tophi reduction may take years. If gout is difficult to control, check patient adherence.

8.4 Colchicine

Colchicine is licensed for use in acute gout and to prevent recurrent attacks.

Mechanism of action

It reduces the inflammatory response to urate crystals, possibly by inhibiting the migration of granulocytes into the inflamed area.

Evidence grading

Grade A evidence for treatment of acute gout (Schlesinger *et al.* 2006).

Preparations

- Tablets (500 micrograms)
- Colchicine can also be given intravenously.

Dosage

For acute gout, 1mg initially, then 500 micrograms every 2–3 hours until pain is relieved or diarrhoea or vomiting occurs, or until a total dose of 6mg is reached. Do not repeat the course of treatment within three days.

For prophylaxis, 500 micrograms two to three times daily.

Side effects

The most common side effects of colchicine involve the stomach and bowel and are dose related. Common side effects include nausea, vomiting, diarrhoea and abdominal pain. Larger doses may cause profuse diarrhoea, gastrointestinal haemorrhage, muscle weakness, skin rashes, renal and hepatic damage. Alopecia, peripheral neuritis and bone marrow depression with agranulocytosis and aplastic anaemia may occur after prolonged treatment.

Cautions

Where profuse diarrhoea may cause serious compromise (for example, in elderly and debilitated patients or those with cardiac, renal, hepatic or gastrointestinal disease).

Interactions

- Colchicine may impair the absorption of vitamin B_{12}.
- May induce muscle disorders when used in combination with ciclosporin.
- Erythromycin, clarithromycin or tolbutamide may lead to colchicine toxicity.

Contra-indications

History of hypersensitivity to colchicine. Blood dyscrasias. Pregnancy and breast-feeding.

Prescribing advice

In those patients with gout where NSAIDs are contra-indicated (see Chapter 5), colchicine can be used. This drug frequently produces abdominal pain and diarrhoea, which can be very difficult for the patient if the gout is already limiting the mobility. These side effects are very prone to occur if the SPC dosage regime is used. Those people who tolerate colchicine learn to take it as soon as the episode starts and sometimes manage to use as little as a 500 micrograms twice-daily regime through the attack. Colchicine should be taken with food.

Monitoring

All patients taking colchicine long-term require full blood count monitoring.

Chapter 9

Corticosteroids

9.1 Overview

Corticosteroids used for rheumatological conditions may be in the form of oral prednisolone, intramuscular or intra-articular methylprednisolone, hydrocortisone or triamcinolone.

When using corticosteroids, be aware that the lowest possible dose for the shortest amount of time will minimise the risks of side effects, particularly osteoporosis. For this reason, parenteral corticosteroids are often used instead of oral corticosteroids.

Once receiving regular corticosteroids for three weeks, adrenal suppression occurs, and in such a situation, if the corticosteroids are stopped abruptly, collapse or death from adrenal insufficiency can occur. (Refer to BNF for most recent guidance: www.bnf.org)

During times of physical stress, increased corticosteroid may be needed and regular corticosteroid may suppress the appropriate response. In this situation, it is important to increase corticosteroids.

9.2 Corticosteroids

Mechanism of action

The precise mechanism by which corticosteroids suppress inflammation is unknown.

Evidence grading

Grade A evidence for oral steroid therapy in establishing control of synovitis and reducing erosion development (Gøtzsche & Johansen 2005; Kirwan *et al.* 2007).

Grade A evidence for intramuscular methylprednisolone controlling synovitis whilst awaiting effects of DMARD therapy in rheumatoid arthritis (RA) (Choy *et al.* 2005; Corkill *et al.* 1990).

Grade A evidence for intra-articular corticosteroids in osteoarthritis and flexor tendon injections (Bellamy *et al.* 2006; Peters-Veluthamaningal *et al.* 2009).

NICE guidance weblink

Rheumatoid arthritis: http://guidance.nice.org.uk/CG79

Preparations

- Tablets, intramuscular injection, intra-articular or intra-synovial injection

Intra-articular methylprednisolone (Depomedrone®) or triamcinolone (Kenalog®) is indicated for local inflammation of joints and soft tissues. Typically 40mg is used for medium-sized joints and 10–20mg for small joints or tendons. For superficial soft tissue injections (for example, for lateral epicondylitis), hydrocortisone is used to minimise the risk of skin atrophy.

Dosage

- Oral prednisolone: 2.5mg (brown) and 5mg (white) or 1mg (white)
- Soluble prednisolone tablets: 5mg
- Intramuscular methylprednisolone: 40mg/ml
- Intra-articular methylprednisolone or triamcinolone: 40mg/ml
- Intra-synovial hydrocortisone: 25mg/ml

Intra-articular methylprednisolone (Depomedrone®) or triamcinolone (Kenalog®) is indicated for local inflammation of joints and soft tissues. Typically 40mg is used for medium-sized joints and 10–20mg for small joints or tendons. For superficial soft tissue injections (for example, for lateral epicondylitis), hydrocortisone is used to minimise the risk of skin atrophy.

Side effects

- Gastrointestinal – dyspepsia, peptic ulceration, nausea
- Musculoskeletal – proximal myopathy, osteoporosis, avascular necrosis
- Endocrine – adrenal suppression, weight gain, increased appetite

- Ophthalmic – glaucoma, corneal or scleral thinning
- Neuropsychiatric effects – euphoria, depression, psychosis
- Other effects – bruising, striae, impaired healing, skin atrophy

Table 9.1: Suggested doses when prescribing corticosteroids

Indication	Oral prednisolone indication	Oral dose range adapted from the British National Formulary 2012
Polymyalgia rheumatica (PMR) and giant cell arteritis (GCA)	✔ ✔	10–15mg daily initially (reduced to 7.5mg for maintenance) 40–60mg initially, followed by maintenance dose of 7.5–10mg daily
Vasculitis polymyositis	✔	60mg initially, followed by maintenance dose of 10–15mg daily
Rheumatoid arthritis	✔	7.5 mg initially, for no longer than 2–4 years

Cautions

Caution is necessary when oral prednisolone is prescribed for patients with a previous history of tuberculosis or X-ray changes characteristic of tuberculosis. Hypertension, congestive heart failure, liver failure, renal insufficiency, diabetes mellitus or osteoporosis. A history of severe affective disorders and particularly those with a previous history of steroid-induced psychoses, epilepsy or seizure disorders, peptic ulceration.

Be aware that suppression of the inflammatory response and immune function increases the susceptibility to infections and their severity. In addition, serious infection (such as septicaemia and tuberculosis) may be masked in patients taking prednisolone.

Contra-indication

Systemic infections.

Interactions

- Drugs such as anti-epileptics, phenytoin and carbamazepine, and rifampicin, rifabutin and primidone may reduce the therapeutic efficacy of prednisolone and other corticosteroids by increasing the rate of metabolism.
- Patients with diabetes mellitus who are receiving insulin and/or oral hypoglycaemic agents may require dosage adjustments to such therapy.
- Salicylates and prednisolone should be used concurrently with caution, and patients receiving both drugs must be observed closely for adverse effects from either drug.
- Erythromycin inhibits metabolism of methylprednisolone and possibly other corticosteroids.
- Response to anticoagulants may be reduced or occasionally enhanced by corticosteroids, and close monitoring of the international normalised ratio (INR) is required.

Prescribing advice

If the patient is going to be referred on to secondary care, discuss initiation of regular corticosteroids with the specialist team first, as clinical, serological and histopathological signs of inflammation will rapidly disappear.

Patients should be advised to carry steroid treatment cards if they receive oral corticosteroids. These cards provide guidance on the precautions to be taken to minimise risk and provide details of prescriber, drug, dosage and duration of treatment.

If a patient is anticipated to be receiving a three-month (or more) course of prednisolone, prevention of corticosteroid induced osteoporosis should be considered.

See: http://www.shef.ac.uk/NOGG/NOGG_Executive_Summary.pdf

The patient's risk factors for osteoporosis can also be entered into a FRAX assessment. The National Osteoporosis Guideline Group (www.shef.ac.uk/NOGG/) gives an overall risk assessment profile for patients and advice on treatment according to the dose of prednisolone prescribed.

Be aware that chickenpox, although normally a minor illness, may be fatal in immunosuppressed patients. Patients without a clear medical history of chickenpox should be advised to avoid close personal contact with chickenpox or herpes zoster and, if exposed, they should seek urgent medical attention. Passive immunisation with varicella zoster immunoglobulin is required for non-immune patients within 10 days of exposure to chicken pox, who are receiving prednisolone or other corticosteroids, or who have taken them within the previous three months. If a diagnosis of chickenpox is confirmed, prednisolone should not be stopped and the dose may need to be increased.

Patients should also be advised to avoid exposure to measles if possible and, if necessary, to seek immediate medical assistance should exposure occur. Intramuscular immunoglobulin prophylaxis may be required.

Intravenous methylprednisolone

This may be used in rheumatology units for an acute flare-up of inflammatory arthritis or induction of remission of vasculitis. It is given to suppress inflammation in cases where lower doses of corticosteroids have not been effective. It is particularly important to screen and treat infection prior to giving the methylprednisolone in this form. Side effects, cautions, contra-indications and interactions are as listed for corticosteroids above.

Evidence grading

Grade A evidence for intravenous methylprednisolone controlling synovitis whilst awaiting effects of methotrexate therapy in rheumatoid arthritis (van der Veen & Bijlsma 1993).

Dosage

Methylprednisolone 1g usually given intravenously on three alternate or consecutive days.

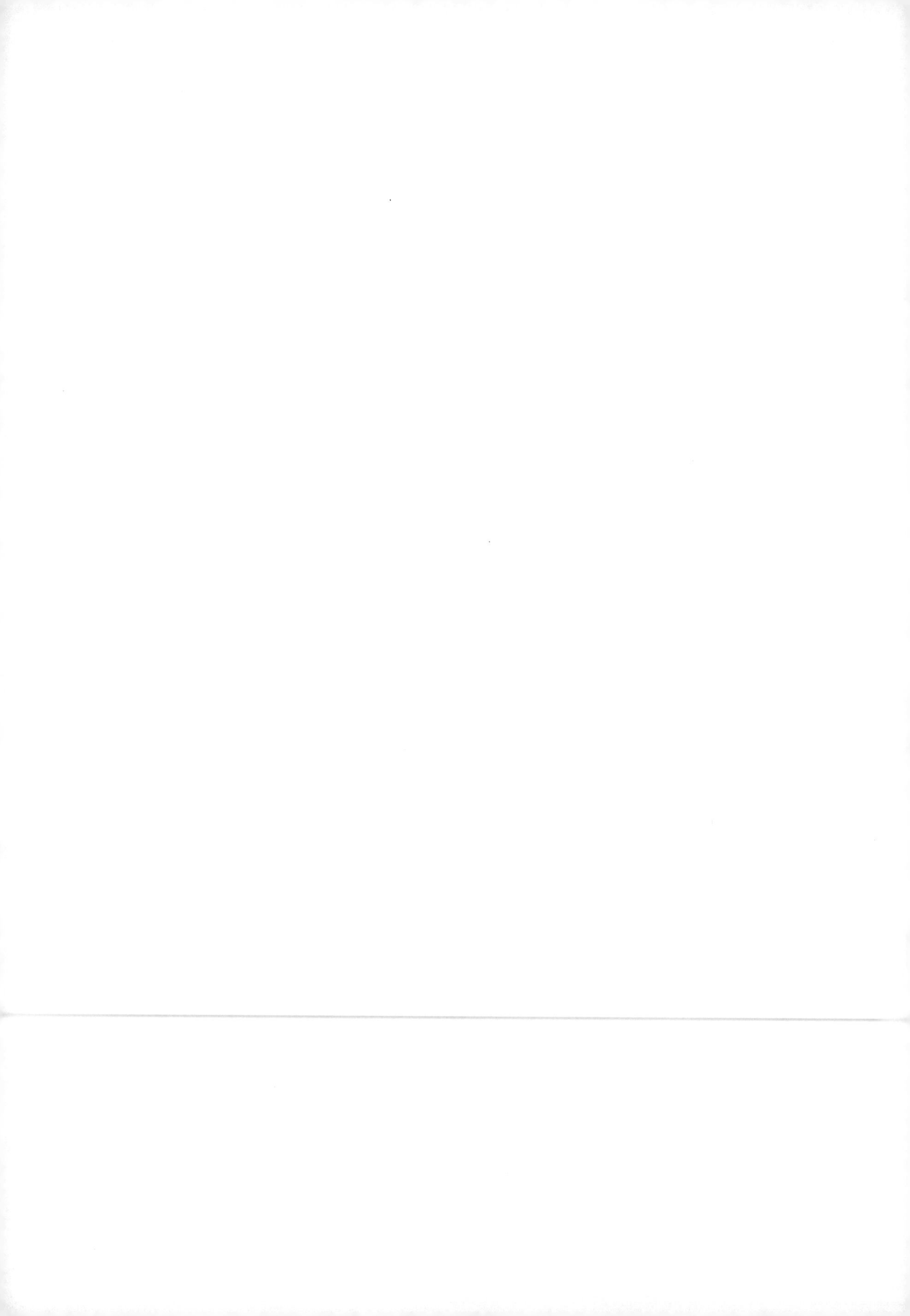

Chapter 10

Case histories

Case 1
Osteoarthritis

For the last 20 years, a 60-year old woman has had episodes, lasting up to eight weeks, of 'losing her spark' with widespread joint aching. She is very frustrated and is feeling anxious about her symptoms. No significant early morning or inactivity stiffness has been reported. There are no other systemic symptoms, past medical history and no relevant family history. She has been a widow for five years, and her anti-depressant was changed three months ago to mirtazapine (15mg daily). She has some sleep disturbance.

On examination, there were some mild osteoarthritis changes in the joints, with particular restriction in movement in the cervical spine and hip. There are no signs of inflammatory arthritis or polymyalgia rheumatica or systemic malignancy. Her erythrocyte sedimentation rate (ESR) has been 31mm/hr, with a normal C-reactive protein (CRP) and other blood tests.

The working diagnosis was inflammatory flares of osteoarthritis. Blood pressure was normal.

There was no help from paracetamol; and ibuprofen and naproxen caused gastrointestinal (GI) side effects.

Consider the following points before reading on.

- **What treatment would you recommend?**
- **Discuss the salient prescribing points.**

Advice

We would suggest that a further try at easing symptoms with a Cox-2 selective non-steroidal anti-inflammatory drug (NSAID) and proton pump inhibitor (PPI) cover is worth considering. It can sometimes take three attempts with an NSAID to find one that suits a patient. In view of the previous GI side effects with ibuprofen and naproxen, we suggest meloxicam (7.5mg daily) with omeprazole (20mg daily). The patient should be counselled on the cardiovascular and GI risks of NSAIDs; to reduce these risks, it's preferable to take them intermittently rather than continuously. Stating this when the initial prescription is provided is very helpful in adjusting the patient's expectations. If available, provide written as well as verbal information about the time it will take for the treatment to work, potential side effects and what to do if they occur.

The prescriber should also consider co-prescription of anti-depressants and NSAIDs. No interaction is reported with mirtazapine (an alpha 2-antagonist anti-depressant) but the commonly used selective serotonin reuptake inhibitors (SSRIs), such as cipramil and fluoxetine, and NSAIDs can both increase risk of peptic ulceration. This may be why the patient did not tolerate the previous NSAIDs. The prescriber needs to weigh up the benefits and risks if an SSRI and NSAID are combined. Co-prescription of a proton pump inhibitor is very important and it must be emphasised that this needs to be taken even in the absence of stomach symptoms.

Because this patient is already on an anti-depressant, co-prescription of a further tricyclic anti-depressant (such as low-dose amitriptyline) would not be considered as a first-line treatment. It may be possible to discuss with the GP whether the current anti-depressant is still needed if the new NSAID is not tolerated. See:

NICE Depression in adults 2009: http://guidance.nice.org.uk/CG90

Review the patient after four weeks, when one would expect the maximal anti-inflammatory effects of the NSAID to be seen, and decide on its effectiveness and continued use. The dose of meloxicam could be increased to 15mg daily if it has only been partially effective. Blood pressure should also be checked at this review appointment.

Case 2
Gout

A 49-year-old man, who had been treated for a calf muscle tear, developed a left knee effusion, which settled with anti-inflammatories. He then developed a severely painful right knee effusion, with erythematous skin changes, and returned to his anti-inflammatories. Both effusions settled, though the erythema at the right knee persisted for a few days. There was no family history of arthritis or other past medical history. He lived with his wife and he was a sales manager in the building industry. He did not smoke, and he drank 40 units of alcohol per week.

A gouty tophi was emerging on the ear and there was some erythema around the right knee. However, the joints were no longer swollen. Blood pressure was normal. The diagnosis was gout. Lifestyle issues and recommendations for people with gout were discussed.

Consider the following points before reading on.

- **What treatment would you recommend?**
- **Discuss the salient prescribing points.**

Advice

We would suggest that he takes his anti-inflammatories for episodes of gout. Naproxen is considered safest so this is recommended as a first-line treatment but sometimes a dose of 500mg three times daily needs to be used, in gout, for the first few days. If this is not effective, diclofenac or etoricoxib may be helpful. (Do not prescribe two NSAIDs together as there is a very high risk of life-threatening GI complications.) Etoricoxib has a 120mg daily seven-day dose for acute attacks of gout.

We would review after two weeks to see if the acute attack has settled and then discuss allopurinol treatment. The patient needs to be committed to taking the treatment in the long term, and to be aware that gout can flare up during the initial months of allopurinol therapy or on stopping it. Hopefully a suitable NSAID will have been found to treat the flare-ups before the allopurinol is started. If necessary, a lower maintenance dose can be given – naproxen 500mg twice daily or etoricoxib 60mg daily. Monitor the patient's blood pressure if etoricoxib is to be used regularly.

Start allopurinol after checking full blood count, renal and liver function tests. If available, provide written as well as verbal information about the time it will take for the treatment to work, the potential side effects and what to do if they occur. Start at 100mg daily, increasing by 100mg increments each month, until uric acid is below 0.36 mmol/l. Once the patient is established on the correct dose of allopurinol, check uric acid levels yearly.

Case 3
Sciatica

This 65-year-old woman had a nine-week history of sciatica in her right leg and was unable to weight bear because of this. Unfortunately, because of the pain she was experiencing, the physiotherapist could only offer a very limited range of treatment modalities. There was no weight loss and no relevant family history. The patient was retired and enjoyed gardening and bowling. She was a cigarette smoker.

Straight leg raising was limited in her right leg to 60 degrees and extension of the lumbar spine reproduced the pain. There was no focal neurology.

Imaging showed degenerative changes only. Blood tests, including renal function, were normal. Clinically, this was lateral recess stenosis from degenerative lumbar spine disease causing sciatica (right 4th lumbar nerve root irritation).

Unfortunately she was unable to tolerate standard analgesics. Tramadol caused vomiting and cocodamol 30/500 caused dizziness and drowsiness. She had tolerated coproxamol in the past but had not been prescribed any.

Consider the following points before reading on.

- **What treatment would you recommend?**
- **Discuss the salient prescribing points.**

Advice

We would suggest that neuropathic medications should be considered. We would start with amitriptyline nocte, 2–4 hours before planned sleep. In view of the patient's age and previous central nervous system side effects with cocodamol, try the lowest dose to begin with (10mg). Advise the patient that this is unlicensed use of the drug (although recommended by NICE for neuropathic pain) and alcohol should be avoided. If available, provide written as well as verbal information about the time it will take for the treatment to work, the potential side effects and what to do if they occur.

Review at two weeks and decide whether to increase fortnightly by 10mg if not too troubled with side effects. If too sedating or anti-cholinergic side effects (such as postural hypotension or dry mouth), try gabapentin. Again, start gabapentin at a low dose (such as 100mg daily) with gradual increase (100mg/week), with regular review. Aim for 300–600mg three times daily for at least three weeks, to see full effects.

If gabapentin is not effective, pregabalin could be considered next. Decide whether to start with 25mg or 75mg nocte, depending on how the patient has tolerated the other drugs.

It is also important to suggest that the physiotherapist should embark on manual physiotherapy, once some effective medication has been found.

Case 4
Osteoporotic fractures (L1/L3)

A 70-year-old man has been found to have three wedge fractures on thoracic spine x-ray. The pain from these fractures has settled. On Dexa scan, his lumbar spine t score was -2.9 and his femoral t-score was -1.9. No cause was found for osteoporosis from the blood test results. It was therefore presumed that features identified in his medical history (previous very high alcohol intake and cigarette smoking and dietary restriction more recently) were contributing to the osteoporosis. When the t-scores were entered into the Sheffield FRAX assessment tool (www.shef.ac.uk/FRAX), the National Osteoporosis Guideline Group (NOGG) algorithm indicated that he was at high risk of future fractures, and treatment should be considered.

Consider the following points before reading on.

- **What treatment would you recommend?**
- **Discuss the salient prescribing points.**

Advice

We would suggest calcium and vitamin D combined supplements, such as Calcichew D3 Forte® (two tablets daily) and a generic bisphosphonate licensed for men, such as alendronate (10mg daily) or risedronate (35 mg weekly).

A study suggested that calcium supplementation might increase the risk of cardiac morbidity. This was somewhat controversial but was widely disseminated (Bolland *et al.* 2010). Following on from this, the national bodies advised that calcium and vitamin D should only be prescribed for patients whose diets were providing insufficient intake of these components. For this individual, 1.2g calcium and 800 IU vitamin D is needed on a daily basis.
See: http://ods.od.nih.gov/factsheets/Calcium-HealthProfessional/

The patient should be counselled on how to take the bisphosphonate to ensure that it is effective (see page 63). This advice always needs to be emphasised and checked at follow-up appointments. If available, provide written as well as verbal information about what the treatment is for, the potential side effects, and what to do if they occur.

Two Medicines and Healthcare Products Regulatory Agency (MHRA) alerts relate to bisphosphonates – the risk of jaw necrosis and atypical femoral fractures. All invasive dental work should be completed prior to commencing bisphosphonate, and good oral hygiene (maintained with regular dental check-ups) should be encouraged when on the treatment. Treatment should be reviewed at five years to see if the ongoing benefit of treatment exceeds the risks of atypical femoral fracture.

It would be important to provide support to the patient to help him stop smoking and continue to drink alcohol only within national recommended limits.

Case 5
Polymyalgia rheumatica

This 77-year-old woman had hypertension, diverticulosis, hiatus hernia and a total knee replacement. She gave a three-month history of wrist pain and swelling, shoulder pain and stiffness, lower back and hamstring pain. She had profound early morning stiffness lasting for hours. Blood tests had shown an elevated ESR at 65mm, and mild anaemia with a haemoglobin 11.1 g/dL. There had been no response to ibuprofen or analgesics. There was no relevant rheumatic family history. She was retired and admitted to drinking 14 units of alcohol per week. Her blood pressure was 130/80.

Clinically there was synovitis at the wrist joints and pain on forced abduction of the shoulder girdle and pelvic girdle. The working diagnosis was polymyalgia rheumatica.

Consider the following points before reading on.

- **What treatment would you recommend?**
- **Discuss the salient prescribing points.**

Advice

The confirmation of the diagnosis would be the miraculous response to corticosteroids. Consensus is with a dose of 15mg of oral prednisolone for two weeks (taken in the mornings). If greater than 75% improvement occurs, the diagnosis of polymyalgia rheumatica is confirmed. Sometimes patients are reluctant to take corticosteroids (often because of concerns over side effects, particularly weight gain) but really at present there is no alternative treatment. If available, provide written as well as verbal information about the time it will take for the treatment to work, the potential side effects, and what to do if they occur.

Once the excellent response to corticosteroids has been seen, a tapering regime for approximately a year to 18 months should be introduced. The easiest regime to remember is 15mg daily for a month, then reduce the dose by 1mg per month. The patient should be given a corticosteroid alert card. We would review the patient regularly to ensure that corticosteroids are being reduced in dose, and inflammatory markers (ESR and CRP) are normal.

Whilst on corticosteroids, the National Osteoporosis Guidance Group (NOGG) has suggested that female patients over the age of 70 years, or with a previous fragility fracture, are all commenced on osteoporosis treatment to prevent osteoporosis if corticosteroid treatment is to be for more than three months. This has recently superseded the Royal College of Physicians 2002 Guidance.

See: http://www.shef.ac.uk/NOGG/NOGG_Executive_Summary.pdf

For younger patients and male patients, osteoporosis risk factors are assessed with a FRAX assessment and possibly a DEXA scan. Treatment is then suggested according to the dose of prednisolone being used.

See: http://www.shef.ac.uk/NOGG/

We would suggest calcium and vitamin D supplementation if the diet is below recommended levels of intake as standard for patients receiving oral corticosteroids. If specific treatment is indicated, daily bisphosphonates are licensed for prevention of corticosteroid osteoporosis in women.

In this case, because of the hiatus hernia, our preference would be for risedronate and a weekly preparation (risedronate 35mg weekly). Risedronate has fewer oesophageal side effects than the other bisphosphonates, and a weekly dosing regime would reduce oesophageal exposure to the bisphosphonate. It would still be important to monitor the patient closely for oesophageal symptoms once they had commenced the risedronate. This would be outside the licensed use so we would inform the GP and patient as to the reasons for this prescription.

The patient should be counselled on how to take the bisphosphonate to ensure that it is effective (see page 63). This advice always needs to be emphasised and checked at follow-up appointments. If available, provide written as well as verbal information about what the treatment is for, the potential side effects, and what to do if they occur.

Case 6
Chronic lumbar spine pain and osteoarthritis

This 64-year-old man gave a two-year history of pain in his lower lumbar spine radiating to the right hip, left ankle and second metacarpophalangeal (MCP) joints. He had previously had physiotherapy, which helped. His symptoms were worse on weight bearing and at work and at the end of the day. He had resisted taking any painkillers in case they made his irritable bowel syndrome flare up. He was now at the point of tears with the pain when walking his dog. There were no inflammatory features to his history. He also had a past history of hypertension and pleural plaques. He worked as an electrical project engineer. He drank less than 14 units of alcohol and did not smoke.

On examination, there were no signs of psoriatic nail disease or inflammatory arthritis. His lumbar spine was tender over the right fourth and fifth facet joint and the pain was worse on extension and extension/rotation. There was tenderness across the left ankle joint line and the second MCP joints.

Blood tests were normal and a pelvic x-ray showed lower lumbar spondylosis and mild osteoarthritis in the right hip.

The diagnosis was degenerative chronic lumbar spine disease (spondylosis) and osteoarthritis as the cause of his pain and there was no association with his psoriasis.

Consider the following points before reading on.

- **What treatment would you recommend?**
- **Discuss the salient prescribing points.**

Advice

In view of his benefits from physiotherapy, we would suggest he takes a further course. As this patient is medication treatment naïve, start at the bottom of the analgesic ladder with over-the-counter paracetamol (1g as required, to a maximum of 4g per day). Suggest that he takes them half an hour before setting off on his walks, as they work better for prevention than when taken at 'breaking point'. Then move to taking them regularly rather than as required.

Suggest adding in NSAIDs. Start with over-the-counter ibuprofen 200–400mg three times daily initially. If ibuprofen does not give sufficient benefit and does not exacerbate his irritable bowel syndrome, prescribe naproxen 250–500mg on an intermittent basis. If available, provide written as well as verbal information about the time it will take for the treatment to work, the potential side effects, and what to do if they occur.

If above treatments are not tolerated or ineffective, try a low-dose tricyclic anti-depressant such as amitriptyline (10mg nocte 2 hours before planned sleep, increasing in 10mg increments every fortnight up, to 50mg if necessary). Counsel that this is an unlicensed use of the drug (although recommended by NICE for chronic back pain) and alcohol should be avoided.

Low-dose tricyclic anti-depressants are suggested as a second-line treatment for irritable bowel syndrome and this may be an attractive option to the patient.

See: NICE Irritable Bowel Syndrome Guideline 2008 http://publications.nice.org.uk/irritable-bowel-syndrome-in-adults-cg61

Review in five weeks' time; amitriptyline could be increased further, up to a maximum dose of 75mg if necessary.

Case 7
Acute prolapsed cervical spine disc

A 41-year-old woman presented with severe right arm pain in C6 distribution, and tingling in the thumb and first finger. There was a nine-week history, following over-extension of her neck during a badminton match. She could not get comfortable, and was not sleeping well. She had initially tried physiotherapy but reported no benefit.

She then tried paracetamol and ibuprofen, which she described as 'not touching the pain'.

Her GP prescribed cocodamol (30/500mg, two to four times a day) and naproxen (500mg, twice a day), and referred her to the spinal clinic. She reported that this combination of medication took the edge off the pain. She experienced no side effects except some constipation but she felt she couldn't reduce the medication and was still struggling with pain control, particularly in the early morning and at the end of the day. There was no significant past medical history, and there was a family history of hypertension.

She smoked at least 20 cigarettes per day, more at present due to pain. She did drink alcohol.

She was very anxious about diagnosis and prognosis and very tearful. She was unable to work because of the pain and reported difficulty in coping with caring for her children.

On examination, cervical spine movements were reduced and there were reduced C6 reflexes on the right and numbness of the thumb. On review of systems, she complained of palpitations. She felt this was because she was getting so anxious and had made an appointment to see her GP about it.

The clinical diagnosis was a prolapsed disc, causing right-sided C6 nerve root compression. A magnetic resonance imaging (MRI) scan of the cervical spine was arranged, as she could need neurosurgical decompression, and pain relief needed to be considered for the next few weeks.

Consider the following points before reading on.

- **What treatment would you recommend?**
- **Discuss the salient prescribing points.**

Advice

Again, we would consider neuropathic medications initially, like gabapentin or pregabalin. We would avoid tricyclic anti-depressants (such as amitriptyline) at this time because of the palpitations, which they may exacerbate – if there is an underlying arrhythmia. The patient seems able to tolerate medications reasonably well and needs rapid pain relief so consider gabapentin (300mg daily), increasing every day by 300mg until 300mg three times daily. Then add in a further 300mg every day until the patient is on 600mg three times daily. Or consider pregabalin (75mg twice daily), doubling every three days to 300mg twice daily. If available, provide written as well as verbal information about the time it will take for the treatment to work, the potential side effects, and what to do if they occur.

Review regularly and slow the regime down if the patient develops troublesome side effects. Review after two weeks of full dose to assess the response. If effective, consider reducing the NSAID, as there is minimal evidence for its efficacy in neuropathic pain and she has a family history of hypertension. If ineffective, withdraw the neuropathic medication as it can cause significant weight gain and exacerbate the situation. Also give advice regarding over-the-counter laxatives and consider splitting paracetamol/codeine and reducing codeine if it is possible to consider reducing the medications.

Case 8
Chronic back pain

This 30-year-old lady was known to have thoracic spine scoliosis. She had her original spinal surgery at the age of 13, and had her surgical spinal rods removed three years ago. Unfortunately none of the surgeries had improved her spinal pain and she was getting inadequate pain control from her current analgesics (tramadol 50mg 1–2 four times daily, pregabalin 300mg twice daily).

For the last six months, she has had a band-like chest pain going all the way round the chest. She has been screened for any underlying respiratory cause for this but the investigations would suggest that there is no respiratory cause. Her scoliosis has been more troublesome since the removal of the rods but she does not want further spinal surgery. The patient feels that tramadol is interfering with her sleeping patterns and causing nightmares, and previously amitriptyline had caused a lot of sedation.

Consider the following points before reading on.

- **What treatment would you recommend?**
- **Discuss the salient prescribing points.**

Advice

We would suggest that her tramadol is withdrawn and she is tried on cocodamol 30/500. This is equivalent strength and may be less stimulatory to her. Pregabalin has not been of any benefit, probably because this is not neuropathic pain, so we would suggest this is withdrawn by 50mg every three days.

Amitriptyline caused drowsiness but there may not be the same problem with nortriptyline or imipramine. Ideally, tricyclic anti-depressants and tramadol should be avoided, as the risk of convulsions is increased. Certainly this combination should not be given to someone with epilepsy or unexplained blackouts. We would therefore suggest waiting until she has been changed over from tramadol to cocodamol before introducing nortriptyline. Start with 10mg 2 hours before planned sleep, and increase in 10mg increments as tolerated up to 50mg. If this is not tolerated, then imipramine (in the same dosage regime) can be tried. Advise the patient that this is an unlicensed use of the drug (although recommended by NICE for chronic back pain) and alcohol should be avoided.

If available, provide written as well as verbal information about the time it will take for the treatment to work, the potential side effects, and what to do if they occur. We would also refer her to the local physiotherapy service to see if they can help with her thoracic spine-related pain.

Case 9
Rheumatoid arthritis

This 69-year-old woman presented with progressive and rapid arthritis occurring over the previous three months. It was affecting the proximal interphalangeal, metacarpophalangeal and wrist joints. There was prolonged early-morning stiffness and little benefit from ibuprofen or naproxen. There was a past medical history of Morton's neuroma, gastro-oesophageal reflux, hypercholesterolaemia and mild chronic obstructive pulmonary disease (COPD). This woman had stopped smoking five years before, and did not drink alcohol. Recently blood tests had shown rheumatoid factor to be three times normal and ESR to be raised at 22mm/hr.

On examination, there was synovitis in the painful joints and the disease activity score was 5.51 (indicating high disease activity). Blood pressure was normal. The diagnosis was early active seropositive rheumatoid arthritis.

Consider the following points before reading on.

- **What treatment would you recommend?**
- **Discuss the salient prescribing points.**

To settle the acute synovitis, we offered corticosteroids, as NSAIDs have been ineffective. We chose methylprednisolone intramuscularly (120mg weekly, on up to three occasions over the next three weeks). If this is difficult to arrange, and the patient is willing to take long-term oral corticosteroids, then prednisolone (at a dose of 7.5mg) would be the alternative option, tapering down and withdrawing once the patient has had two years of treatment. If available, provide written as well as verbal information about the time it will take for the treatment to work, the potential side effects, and what to do if they occur.

Prophylaxis against osteoporosis would also need to be considered if the patient has more than three months of oral prednisolone.

Methotrexate, in combination with another disease-modifying anti-rheumatic drug (DMARD), is recommended by NICE if there is no contra-indication.

We arranged for spirometry and a chest x-ray, as well as recent full blood count, renal function and liver function tests. The results were satisfactory and visual acuity with reading glasses was found to be normal. Methotrexate (10mg orally weekly), folic acid (5mg weekly) and hydroxychloroquine (200mg twice daily) were commenced after counselling and arranging blood test monitoring locally, according to the British Society of Rheumatology (BSR) guidance (Chakravarty *et al.* 2008).

See: http://rheumatology.oxfordjournals.org/content/47/6/924.full.pdf+html

Annual eye checks from the optician were recommended. We suggest providing written as well as verbal information about the time it will take for the treatment to work, the potential side effects, and what to do if they occur.

An important point to consider is whether methotrexate can be safely prescribed for patients with COPD. Methotrexate has a rare side effect of pneumonitis, and several studies have been undertaken to find out if it is possible to predict which patients will develop this complication. Unfortunately this has not been consistently established. It is therefore safest to assume that all patients could develop pneumonitis and educate them carefully on the warning signs (progressive shortness of breath and cough). Pragmatically, spirometry provides a quick test that can assess lung volumes and whether reasonable capacity exists to survive this complication, assuming that pneumonitis is picked up early. We take a cut-off of 1 litre (Sathi *et al.* 2012).

A patient who has repeated exacerbations of breathlessness may be difficult to establish on methotrexate. However, a patient with mild lung disease and well-preserved lung volumes can be offered methotrexate.

Appendix

List of common proprietary names

Non-proprietary	Proprietary
Alendronic acid	Fosamax
Allopurinol	Zyloric
Buprenorphine	Patches: Butrans, Transtec
Calcium and vitamin D	Accrete D3, Adcal-D3, Cacit D3, Calceos, Calcichew D3 Forte, Calcovit D3, Sandocal+D
Capsaicin	Zacin, Axsain
Celecoxib	Celebrex
Codeine plus paracetamol	Codipar, Kapake, Solpadol, Tylex
Denosumab	Prolia
Diclofenac	Voltarol, Diclomax, Dicloflex
Duloxetine hydrochloride	Cymbalta
Etoracoxib	Arcoxia
Febuxostat	Adenuric
Fentanyl	Patches: Durogesic Dtrans

Gabapentin	Neurontin
Hydrocortisone	Parenteral preps: Efcortesol, Solu-Cortel
Hydroxychloroquine	Plaquenil
Ibandronic acid	Bondronat, Bonviva
Ibuprofen	Brufen
Leflunomide	Arava
Lidocaine	Plasters: Versastis
Methotrexate	Parenteral preps: Ebetrex, Metoject
Methylprednisolone	Medrone Parenteral preps; Solu-medrone, Depo-medrone
Morphine	Solutions: Oramorph Tablets: Sevredol Modified release 12-hrly preps: Filnarine, Morphgesic, MST Continus, Zomorph Modified release 24-hrly preps: MXL
Naproxen	Naprosyn, Synflex
Nortriptyline	Allegron
Oxycodone	Oxynorm Modified release: Oxycontin
Paracetamol	Panadol
Pregabalin	Lyrica
Raloxifene	Evista
Risedronate	Actonel
Strontium ranelate	Protelos
Sulfasalazine	Salazopyrin
Teriparatide	Forsteo

Tramadol	Zamadol, Zydol Modified release 12-hrly preps: Larapam, Mabron, Marol, Maxitram, Tramquel, Zamadol, Zeridame, Zydol Modified release 24-hrly preps: Tradorec, Zamadol, Zydol
Triamcinolone	Kenalog
Zoledronic acid	Aclasta

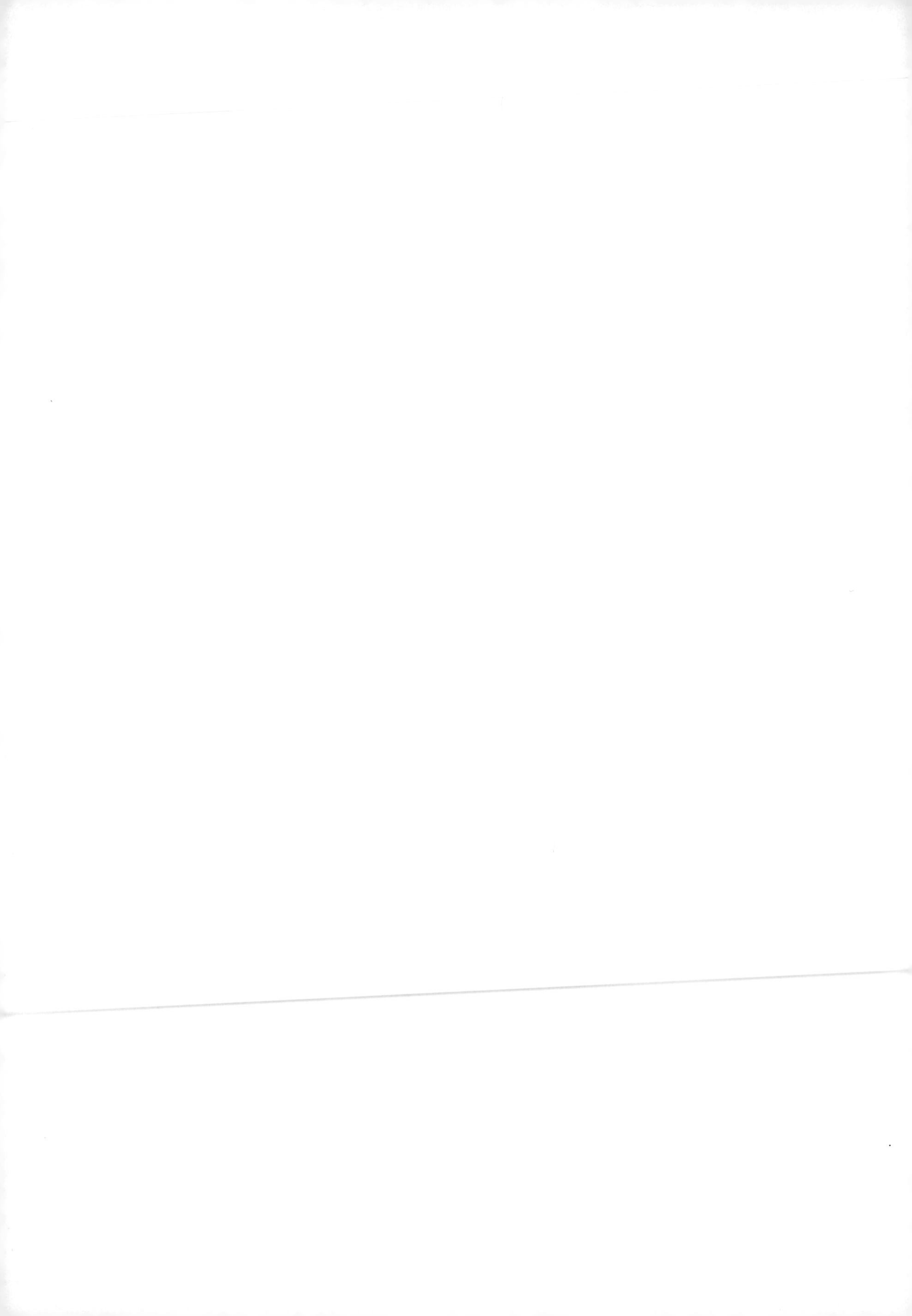

References

Arnold, L.M., Rosen, A., Pritchett, Y.L., D'Souza, D.N., Goldstein, D.J., Iyengar, S. & Wernicke, J.F. (2005). A randomized, double-blind, placebo-controlled trial of duloxetine in the treatment of women with fibromyalgia with or without major depressive disorder. *Pain.* **119** (1–3), 5–15.

Avenell, A., Gillespie, W.J., Gillespie, L.D. & O'Connell, D. (2009). Vitamin D and vitamin D analogues for preventing fractures associated with involutional and post-menopausal osteoporosis. Cochrane Database of Systematic Reviews, Issue 2. Art. No.: CD000227. DOI: 10.1002/14651858.CD000227.pub3.

Barber, N., Parsons, J., Clifford, S., Darracott, R. & Horne, R. (2004). Patients' problems with new medication for chronic conditions. *Quality and Safety in Health Care.* **13**, 172–75.

Bellamy, N., Campbell, J., Welch, V., Gee, T.L., Bourne, R. & Wells, G.A. (2006). Intraarticular corticosteroid for treatment of osteoarthritis of the knee. Cochrane Database of Systematic Reviews, Issue 2. Art. No.: CD005328. DOI: 10.1002/14651858.CD005328.pub2.

Bennett, R.M., Kamin, M., Karim, R. & Rosenthal, N. (2003). Tramadol and acetaminophen combination tablets in the treatment of fibromyalgia pain: a double-blind, randomized, placebo-controlled study. *American Journal of Medicine.* **114** (7), 537–45.

Bianchi, G., Czerwinski, E., Kenwright, A., Burdeska, A., Recker, R.R., Felsenberg, D., Ringe, J.D. & Doherty, J.G. (2012). Long-term administration of quarterly IV ibandronate is effective and well tolerated in post-menopausal osteoporosis: 5-year data from the DIVA study long-term extension. *Osteoporosis International.* **23** (6), 1769–78.

Bolland, M.J., Avenell, A., Baron, J.A., Grey, A., MacLennan, G.S., Gamble, G.D. & Reid, I.R. (29 July 2010). Effect of calcium supplements on risk of myocardial infarction and cardiovascular events: meta-analysis. *British Medical Journal.* **341**, c3691.

British Pain Society (2010). 'Opioids for persistent pain: Good practice.' http://www.britishpainsociety.org/book_opioid_main.pdf

Cepeda, M.S., Camargo, F., Zea, C. & Valencia, L. (2006). Tramadol for osteoarthritis. Cochrane Database of Systematic Reviews, Issue 3. Art. No.: CD005522. DOI: 10.1002/14651858.CD005522.pub2.

Caulfield, H. (2004). Responsibility, accountability and liability in nurse prescribing. *Prescribing Nurse.* **2** (2), 18–21.

Chakravarty, K., McDonald, H., Pullar, T., Taggart, A., Chalmers, R., Oliver, S., Mooney, J., Somerville, M., Bosworth, A. & Kennedy, T. (2008). *BSR/BHPR guideline for disease-modifying anti-rheumatic drug (DMARD) therapy in consultation with the British Association of Dermatologists. Rheumatology* (Oxford, England). **47** (6), 924–25.

Challapalli, V., Tremont-Lukats, I.W., McNicol, E.D., Lau, J. & Carr, D.B. (2005). Systemic administration of local anesthetic agents to relieve neuropathic pain. Cochrane Database of Systematic Reviews, Issue 4. Art. No.: CD003345. DOI: 10.1002/14651858.CD003345.pub2.

Chikura, B., Lane, S. & Dawson, J.K. (2009). *Clinical expression of leflunomide-induced pneumonitis. Rheumatology* (Oxford, England). **48** (9), 1065–68.

Choy, E.H., Kingsley, G.H., Khoshaba, B., Pipitone, N. & Scott, D.L. (2005). A two year randomised controlled trial of intramuscular depot steroids in patients with established rheumatoid arthritis who have shown an incomplete response to disease modifying antirheumatic drugs. *Annals of the Rheumatic Diseases.* **64** (9), 1288–93.

Cobra, C.J., Cobra, J.F. & Cobra, N.C. (1983). Use of piroxicam in the treatment of acute gout. *European Journal of Rheumatology and Inflammation.* **6** (1), 126–33.

Corkill, M.M., Kirkham, B.W., Chikanza, I.C., Gibson, T. & Panayi, G.S. (1990). Intramuscular depot methylprednisolone induction of chrysotherapy in rheumatoid arthritis: a 24-week randomized controlled trial. *British Journal of Rheumatology.* **29**, (4), 274–79.

de Craen, A.J., Di Giulio, G., Lampe-Schoenmaeckers, J.E., Kessels, A.G. & Kleijnen, J. (1996). Analgesic efficacy and safety of paracetamol-codeine combinations versus paracetamol alone: a systematic review. *British Medical Journal*. **313** (7053), 321–25.

Department of Health (2006). *Improving patients' access to medicines: A guide to implementing nurse and pharmacist independent prescribing within the NHS in England.* http://www.dh.gov.uk/prod_consum_dh/groups/dh_digitalassets/@dh/@en/documents/digitalasset/dh_4133747.pdf

Derry, S., Lloyd, R., Moore, R.A. & McQuay, H.J. (2009). Topical capsaicin for chronic neuropathic pain in adults. Cochrane Database of Systematic Reviews, Issue 4. Art. No.: CD007393. DOI: 10.1002/14651858.CD007393.pub2.

Derry, S., Moore, R.A. & Rabbie, R. (2012). Topical NSAIDs for chronic musculoskeletal pain in adults. Cochrane Database of Systematic Reviews, Issue 9. Art. No.: CD007400. DOI: 10.1002/14651858.CD007400.pub2.

Deshpande, A., Furlan, A.D., Mailis-Gagnon, A., Atlas, S. & Turk, D. (2007). Opioids for chronic low-back pain. Cochrane Database of Systematic Reviews, Issue 3. Art. No.: CD004959. DOI: 10.1002/14651858.CD004959.pub3.

Duehmke, R.M., Hollingshead, J. & Cornblath, D.R. (2006). Tramadol for neuropathic pain. Cochrane Database of Systematic Reviews, Issue 3. Art. No.: CD003726. DOI: 10.1002/14651858.CD003726.pub3.

Eckhardt, K., Li, S., Ammon, S., Schanzle, G., Mikus, G. & Eichelbaum, M. (1998). Same incidence of adverse drug events after codeine administration irrespective of the genetically determined differences in morphine formation. *Pain*. **76**, (1–2), 27–33.

Eisenberg, E., McNicol, E.D. & Carr, D.B. (2006). Opioids for neuropathic pain. Cochrane Database of Systematic Reviews, Issue 3. Art. No.: CD006146. DOI: 10.1002/14651858.CD00614.

Furlan, A.D., Sandoval, J.A., Mailis-Gagnon, A. & Tunks, E. (2006). Opioids for chronic noncancer pain: a meta-analysis of effectiveness and side effects. *Canadian Medical Association Journal*. **174** (11), 1589–94.

Gaujoux-Viala, C., Smolen, J.S., Landewé, R., Dougados, M., Kvien, T.K., Mola, E.M., Scholte-Voshaar, M., van Riel, P. & Gossec, L. (2010). Current evidence for the management of rheumatoid arthritis with synthetic disease-modifying antirheumatic drugs: a systematic literature review informing the EULAR recommendations for the management of rheumatoid arthritis. *Annals of the Rheumatic Diseases*. **69** (6), 1004–09.

Golicki, D., Niewada, M., Lis, J., Pol, K., Hermanowski, T. & Tlustochowicz, M. (2012). Leflunomide in monotherapy of rheumatoid arthritis: meta-analysis of randomized trials. *Archives of Internal Medicine*. **122** (1–2), 22–31.

Gøtzsche, P.C. & Johansen, H.K. (2005). Short-term low-dose corticosteroids vs placebo and nonsteroidal antiinflammatory drugs in rheumatoid arthritis. Cochrane Database of Systematic Reviews, Issue 1. Art. No.: CD000189. DOI: 10.1002/14651858.CD000189.pub2.

Han, S.L. & Wan, S.L. (2012). Effect of teriparatide on bone mineral density and fracture in post-menopausal osteoporosis: meta-analysis of randomised controlled trials. *International Journal of Clinical Practice*. **66** (2), 199–209.

Harris, S.T., Blumentals, W.A., Miller, P.D., Papapoulos, S., Chapurlat, R., Libanati, C., Brandi, M.L., Brown, J.P., Czerwinski, E., Krieg, M.A., Man, Z., Mellstrom, D., Radominski, S.C., Reginster, J.Y., Resch, H., Ivorra, J., Roux, C., Vittinghoff, E., Austin, M., Daizadeh, N., Bradley, M.N., Grauer, A., Cummings, S.R. & Bone, H.G. (2008). Ibandronate and the risk of non-vertebral and clinical fractures in women with post-menopausal osteoporosis: results of a meta-analysis of phase III studies. *Current Medical Research and Opinion*. **24** (1), 237–45

Häuser, W., Urrútia, G., Tort, S., Üçeyler, N. & Walitt, B. (2013). Serotonin and noradrenaline reuptake inhibitors (SNRIs) for fibromyalgia syndrome. Cochrane Database of Systematic Reviews, Issue 1. Art. No: CD010292. DOI: 10.1002/14651858.CD010292

Häuser, W., Wolfe, F., Tölle, T., Uçeyler, N. & Sommer, C. (2012). The role of anti-depressants in the management of fibromyalgia syndrome: a systematic review and meta-analysis. *CNS Drugs*. **26** (4), 297–307.

Health and Care Professionals Council (2012). Standards of conduct, performance and ethics: http://www.hpcuk.org/assets/documents/10003B6EStandardsof conduct,performanceandethics.pdf

Health and Care Professionals Council (2013). Standards for prescribing: http://www.hpc-uk.org/assets/documents/10004160Standardsforprescribing.pdf

Hochberg, M.C., Wohlreich, M., Gaynor, P., Hanna, S. & Risser, R. (2012). Clinically relevant outcomes based on analysis of pooled data from 2 trials of duloxetine in patients with knee osteoarthritis. *Journal of Rheumatology*. **39** (2), 352–58.

Jansen, J.P., Gert J.D. Bergman, Huels, J., Olson, M., Harris, S.T., Blumentals, W.A., Miller, P.D., Papapoulos, S., Chapurlat, R., Libanati, C., Brandi, M.L., Brown, J.P., Czerwinski, E., Krieg, M.A., Man, Z., Mellstrom, D., Radominski, S.C., Reginster, J.Y., Resch, H., Ivorra, J., Roux, C., Vittinghoff, E., Austin, M., Daizadeh, N., Bradley, M.N., Grauer, A., Cummings, S.R. & Bone, H.G. (2012). Osteoporosis: The efficacy of bisphosphonates in the prevention of vertebral, hip, and nonvertebral- non hip fractures in osteoporosis: a network meta-analysis. *Seminars in Arthritis and Rheumatism*. **40** (4), 275–84.

Jones, G., Crotty, M. & Brooks, P. (2000). Interventions for treating psoriatic arthritis. Cochrane Database of Systematic Reviews, Issue 3. Art. No.: CD000212. DOI: 10.1002/14651858.CD000212

Jordan, K.M., Cameron, J.S., Snaith, M., Zhang, W., Doherty, M., Seckl, J., Hingorani, A., Jaques, R. & Nuki, G. (2007). British Society for Rheumatology and British Health Professionals in Rheumatology guideline for the management of gout. *Rheumatology*. **46**, 1372–74.

Kanis, J.A., Johansson, H., Oden, A., McCloskey, E.V., Bianchi, G., Czerwinski, E., Kenwright, A., Burdeska, A., Recker, R.R., Felsenberg, D., Ringe, J.D. & Doherty, J.G. (2010). A meta-analysis of the efficacy of raloxifene on all clinical and vertebral fractures and its dependency on FRA (R). *Bone*. **47** (4), 729–35.

Khaliq, W., Alam, S. & Puri, N.K. (2007). Topical lidocaine for the treatment of postherpetic neuralgia. Cochrane Database of Systematic Reviews, Issue 2. Art. No.: CD004846. DOI: 10.1002/14651858.CD004846.pub2.

Kirwan, J.R., Bijlsma, J.W.J., Boers, M. & Shea, B. (2007). Effects of glucocorticoids on radiological progression in rheumatoid arthritis. Cochrane Database of Systematic Reviews, Issue 1. Art. No.: CD006356. DOI: 10.1002/14651858.CD006356

Knevel, R., Schoels, M., Huizinga, T., Aletaha, D., Burmester, G.R., Combe, B., Landewe, R.B., Smolen, J.S., Sokka, T. & van der Heidje, D.M. (2010). Current evidence for a strategic approach to the management of rheumatoid arthritis with disease-modifying antirheumatic drugs: a systematic literature review informing the EULAR recommendations for the management of rheumatoid arthritis. *Annals of the Rheumatic Diseases*. **69** (6), 976–86.

Kosuwon, W., Sirichatiwapee, W., Wisanuyotin, T., Jeeravipoolvarn, P. & Laupattarakasem, W. (2010). Efficacy of symptomatic control of knee osteoarthritis with 0.0125% of capsaicin versus placebo. *Journal of the Medical Association of Thailand (Chotmaihet thangphaet)*. **93** (10), 1188–95.

Kuffner, E.K., Temple, A.R., Cooper, K.M., Baggish, J.S. & Parenti, D.L. (2006). Retrospective analysis of transient elevations in alanine aminotransferase during long-term treatment with acetaminophen in osteoarthritis clinical trials. *Current Medical Research and Opinion*. **22**, 11, 2137–48.

Langford, R., McKenna, F., Ratcliffe, S., Vojtassak, J. & Richarz, U. (2006). Transdermal fentanyl for improvement of pain and functioning in osteoarthritis: a randomized, placebo-controlled trial. *Arthritis and Rheumatism Journal*. **54** (6), 1829–37.

Levy, R.A., Vilela, V.S., Cataldo, M.J., Ramos, R.C., Duarte, J.L., Tura, B.R., Albuquerque, E.M. & Jesus, N.R. (2001). Hydroxychloroquine (HCQ) in lupus pregnancy: double-blind and placebo-controlled study. *Lupus*. **10** (6), 401–04.

Lunn, M.P.T., Hughes, R.A.C. & Wiffen, P.J. (2009). Duloxetine for treating painful neuropathy or chronic pain. Cochrane Database of Systematic Reviews, Issue 4. Art. No.: CD007115. DOI: 10.1002/14651858.CD007115.pub2.

Luqmani, R., Hennell, S., Estrach, C., Birrell, F., Bosworth, A., Davenport, G., Fokke, C., Goodson, N., Jeffreson, P., Lamb, E., Mohammed, R., Oliver, S., Stableford, Z., Walsh, D., Washbrook, C. & Webb, F. (13 July 2006). British Society for Rheumatology and British Health Professionals in Rheumatology Guideline for the Management of Rheumatoid Arthritis (The first 2 years). *Rheumatology* (Oxford). **45** (9), 1167–9.

Madhok, R., Wu, O., McKellar, G. & Singh, G. (2006). Non-steroidal anti-inflammatory drugs – changes in prescribing may be warranted. *Rheumatology* (Oxford). **45** (12), 1458–60.

Manchikanti, L., Vallejo, R., Manchikanti, K.N., Benyamin, R.M., Datta, S. & Christo, P.J. (2011). Effectiveness of long-term opioid therapy for chronic non-cancer pain. *Pain Physician.* **14** (2), E133–56.

Mason, L., Moore, R.A., Derry, S., Edwards, J.E. & McQuay, H.J. (2004a). Systematic review of topical capsaicin for the treatment of chronic pain. *British Medical Journal.* **328** (7446), 991.

Massey, T., Derry, S., Moore, R.A. & McQuay, H.J. (2010) Topical NSAIDs for acute pain in adults. Cochrane Database of Systematic Reviews, Issue 6. Art. No.: CD007402. DOI: 10.1002/14651858.CD007402.pub2.

McGettigan, P. & Henry, D. (2011). Cardiovascular risk with non-steroidal anti-inflammatory drugs: systematic review of population-based controlled observational studies. *PLOS Medicine.* **8** (9), e1001098–e1001098.

McQuay, H.J., Carroll, D. & Glynn, C.J. (1992). Low dose amitriptyline in the treatment of chronic pain. *Anaesthesia.* **47** (8), 646–52.

Meeus, M. & Nijs, J. (2007). Central sensitization: a biopsychosocial explanation for chronic widespread pain in patients with fibromyalgia and chronic fatigue syndrome. *Clinical Rheumatology.* **26** (4), 465–73.

Misuse of Drugs (Amendment No. 2) (England, Wales and Scotland) Regulations 2012.

Miller, P.D., Brown, J.P., Siris, E.S., Hoseyni, M.S., Axelrod, D.W. & Bekker, P.J. (1999). A randomized, double-blind comparison of risedronate and etidronate in the treatment of Paget's disease of bone. Paget's Risedronate/Etidronate Study Group. *American Journal of Medicine.* **106** (5), 513.

Moore, A., Collins, S., Carroll, D. & McQuay, H. (1997). Paracetamol with and without codeine in acute pain: a quantitative systematic review. *Pain.* **70** (2–3), 193–201.

Moore, R.A., Derry, S., Aldington, D., Cole, P. & Wiffen, P.J. (2012). Amitriptyline for neuropathic pain and fibromyalgia in adults. Cochrane Database of Systematic Reviews, Issue 12. Art. No.: CD008242. DOI: 10.1002/14651858.CD008242.pub2.

Moore, R.A., Derry, S., McQuay, H.J. & Wiffen, P.J. (2011a). Single dose oral analgesics for acute postoperative pain in adults. Cochrane Database of Systematic Reviews, Issue 9. Art. No.: CD008659. DOI: 10.1002/14651858.CD008659.pub2.

Moore, R.A., Straube, S., Wiffen, P.J., Derry, S. & McQuay, H.J. (2009). Pregabalin for acute and chronic pain in adults. Cochrane Database of Systematic Reviews, Issue 3. Art. No.: CD007076. DOI: 10.1002/14651858.CD007076.pub2.

Moore, R.A., Wiffen, P.J., Derry, S. & McQuay, H.J. (2011b). Gabapentin for chronic neuropathic pain and fibromyalgia in adults. Cochrane Database of Systematic Reviews, Issue 3. Art. No.: CD007938. DOI: 10.1002/14651858.CD007938.pub2.

National Osteoporosis Guideline Group (2013) Osteoporosis – Clinical guideline for prevention and treatment of osteoporosis: http://www.shef.ac.uk/NOGG/NOGG_Executive_Summary.pdf

National Prescribing Centre (2012). A single competency framework for all practitioners: http://www.npc.co.uk/improving_safety/improving_quality/resources/single_comp_framework.pdf

NICE (2008a). Ankylosing spondylitis – adalimumab, etanercept and infliximab TA143: http://guidance.nice.org.uk/TA143

NICE (2011a). Ankylosing spondylitis – golimumab TA233: http://guidance.nice.org.uk/TA233

NICE (2009a). Depression in adults CG90: http://guidance.nice.org.uk/CG90

NICE (2012b). Headaches: Diagnosis and management of headaches in young people and adults. http://publications.nice.org.uk/headaches-cg150/guidance.

NICE (2008b). Hyperuricaemia-Febuxostat. Febuxostat for the management of Hyperuricaemia in people with gout TA164: http://guidance.nice.org.uk/TA164

NICE (2008c). Irritable bowel syndrome in adults: Diagnosis and management of irritable bowel syndrome in primary care CG61: http://publications.nice.org.uk/irritable-bowel-syndrome-in-adults-cg61

NICE (2009b). Low Back pain – Early management of persistent non-specific low back pain CG 88: http://guidance.nice.org.uk/CG88

NICE (2009c). Medicines adherence: Involving patients in decisions about prescribed medicines and supporting adherence CG76: http://publications.nice.org.uk/medicines-adherence-cg76

NICE (2008d). Osteoarthritis: The care and managements of osteoarthritis in adults CG59: http://guidance.nice.org.uk/CG59

NICE (2010b). Neuropathic pain – pharmacological management CG96: http://guidance.nice.org.uk/CG96

NICE (2010a). Osteoporotic fractures – Denosumab TA204: http://guidance.nice.org.uk/TA204

NICE (2011b). Osteoporosis: Primary prevention of osteoporosis TA160: http://guidance.nice.org.uk/TA160

NICE (2011c). Osteoporosis: Secondary prevention of osteoporosis TA161: http://guidance.nice.org.uk/TA161

NICE (2012a). Osteoporosis: assessing the risk of fragility fracture CG141: http://www.nice.org.uk/CG146

NICE (2010). Psoriatic arthritis – etanercept, infliximab and adalimumab TA199: http://guidance.nice.org.uk/TA199

NICE (2007). Rheumatoid arthritis – adalimumab, etanercept and infliximab TA130: http://guidance.nice.org.uk/TA130

NICE (2009d). Rheumatoid arthritis: the management of rheumatoid arthritis in adults CG79: http://guidance.nice.org.uk/CG79

Noble, M., Treadwell, J.R., Tregear, S.J., Coates, V.H., Wiffen, P.J., Akafomo, C. & Schoelles, K.M. (2010). Long-term opioid management for chronic noncancer pain. Cochrane Database of Systematic Reviews, Issue 1. Art. No.: CD006605. DOI: 10.1002/14651858.CD006605.pub2.

Nursing and Midwifery Council (2006). Standards of proficiency for nurse and midwife prescribers: http://www.nmc-uk.org/Documents/NMC-Publications/NMC- Standards-proficiency-nurse-and-midwife-prescribers.pdf

O'Dell, J.R., Leff, R., Paulsen, G., Haire, C., Mallek, J., Eckhoff, P.J., Fernandez, A., Blakely, K., Wees, S., Stoner, J., Hadley, S., Felt, J., Palmer, W., Waytz, P., Churchill, M., Klassen, L. & Moore, G. (2002). Treatment of rheumatoid arthritis with methotrexate and hydroxychloroquine, methotrexate and sulfasalazine, or a combination of the three medications: results of a two-year, randomized, double-blind, placebo-controlled trial. *Arthritis and Rheumatism*. **46** (5), 1164–70.

O'Donnell, S., Cranney, A., Wells, G.A., Adachi, J. & Reginster, J.Y. (2006). Strontium ranelate for preventing and treating post-menopausal osteoporosis. Cochrane Database of Systematic Reviews, Issue 4. Art.No.: CD005326. DOI: 10.1002/14651858.CD005326.pub3.

Osiri, M., Shea, B., Robinson, V., Suarez-Almazor, M., Strand, V., Tugwell, P. & Wells, G. (2003). Leflunomide for the treatment of rheumatoid arthritis: a systematic review and metaanalysis. *Journal of Rheumatology.* **30** (6), 1182–90.

Papapoulos, S., Chapurlat, R., Libanati, C., Brandi, M.L., Brown, J.P., Czerwinski, E., Krieg, M.A., Man, Z., Mellstrom, D., Radominski, S.C., Reginster, J.Y., Resch, H., Ivorra, J., Roux, C., Vittinghoff, E., Austin, M., Daizadeh, N., Bradley, M.N., Grauer, A., Cummings, S.R. & Bone, H.G. (2012). Five years of denosumab exposure in women with post-menopausal osteoporosis: Results from the first two years of the FREEDOM extension. *Journal of Bone and Mineral Research.* **27** (3), 694–701.

Peters-Veluthamaningal, C., van der Windt, D.A.W.M., Winters, J.C. & Meyboom-de Jong, B. (2009). Corticosteroid injection for trigger finger in adults. Cochrane Database of Systematic Reviews, Issue 1. Art. No.: CD005617. DOI: 10.1002/14651858.CD005617.pub2.

Reid, I.R., Miller, P. & Lyles, K. (2005). Comparison of a single infusion of zoledronic acid with risedronate for Paget's disease. *New England Journal of Medicine.* **353**, 898–908.

Reginster, J.Y., Kaufman, J.M., Goemaere, S., Devogelaer, J.P., Benhamou, C.L., Felsenberg, D., Diaz-Curiel, M., Brandi, M.L., Badurski, J., Wark, J., Balogh, A., Bruyere, O., Roux, C., Kanis, J.A., Johansson, H., Oden, A. & McCloskey, E.V. (2012). Maintenance of antifracture efficacy over 10 years with strontium ranelate in post-menopausal osteoporosis. *Osteoporosis International.* **23** (3), 1115–22.

Ringe, J.D. & Doherty, J.G. (2010). Absolute risk reduction in osteoporosis: assessing treatment efficacy by number needed to treat. *Rheumatology International.* **30** (7), 863–69.

Roelofs, P.D.D.M., Deyo, R.A., Koes, B.W., Scholten, R.J.P.M. & van Tulder, M.W. (2008). Non-steroidal anti-inflammatory drugs for low back pain. Cochrane Database of Systematic Reviews, Issue 1. Art. No.: CD000396. DOI: 10.1002/14651858.CD000396.pub3.

Royal Pharmaceutical Society of Great Britain (2012). *Medicine, Ethics and Practice, The professional guide for pharmacists*. Edition 36.

Sathi, N., Chikura, B., Kaushik, V.V., Wiswell, R. & Dawson, J.K. (2012). How common is methotrexate pneumonitis? A large prospective study investigates. *Clinical Rheumatology.* **31** (1), 79–83.

Saarto, T. & Wiffen, P.J. (2007). Anti-depressants for neuropathic pain. Cochrane Database of Systematic Reviews, Issue 4. Art. No.: CD005454. DOI: 10.1002/14651858.CD005454.pub2.

Schlesinger, N., Schumacher, R., Catton, M. & Maxwell, L. (2006). Colchicine for acute gout. Cochrane Database of Systematic Reviews. no. 4, p. CD006190.

Schumacher, H.R., Jr., Boice, J.A., Daikh, D.I., Mukhopadhyay, S., Malmstrom, K., Ng, J., Tate, G.A. & Molina, J. (2002). Randomised double blind trial of etoricoxib and indometacin in treatment of acute gouty arthritis. *British Medical Journal.* **324** (7352), 1488–92.

Schumacher, H.R., Becker, M.A., Wortmann, R.L., MacDonald, P.A., Hunt, B., Streit, J., Lademacher, C. & Joseph-Ridge, N. (2008). Effects of febuxostat versus allopurinol and placebo in reducing serum urate in subjects with hyperuricemia and gout: A 28-week, phase III, randomized, double-blind, parallel-group trial. *Arthritis and Rheumatism – arthritis care and research.* **59** (11), 1540–48.

Shi, W., Yong, M.W., Li, S.L., Yan, M., Li, D., Neng, N.C. & Bin, Y.C. (2004). Safety and efficacy of oral nonsteroidal anti-inflammatory drugs in patients with rheumatoid arthritis. *Clinical Drug Investigation.* **24** (2), 89–101.

Sorge, J. & Sittl, R. (2004). Transdermal buprenorphine in the treatment of chronic pain: results of a phase III, multicenter, randomized, double-blind, placebo-controlled study. *Clinical Therapy.* **26** (11), 1808–20.

Steiner, D.J., Sitar, S., Wen, W., Sawyer, G., Munera, C., Ripa, S.R. & Landau, C. (2011). Efficacy and safety of the seven-day buprenorphine transdermal system in opioid-naïve patients with moderate to severe chronic low back pain: an enriched, randomized, double-blind, placebo-controlled study. *Journal of Pain and Symptom Management.* **42**, 903–17.

Stevenson, M., Davis, S., Lloyd-Jones, M. & Beverley, C. (2007). The clinical effectiveness and cost-effectiveness of strontium ranelate for the prevention of osteoporotic fragility fractures in post-menopausal women. *Health Technology Assessment.* **11** (4), 1–134.

Suarez-Almazor, M.E., Belseck, E., Shea, B., Homik, J., Wells, G. & Tugwell, P. (2000a). Antimalarials for treating rheumatoid arthritis. Cochrane Database of Systematic Reviews. no. 4, p. CD000959.

Suarez-Almazor, M.E., Belseck, E., Shea, B., Wells, G .& Tugwell, P. (1998a). Methotrexate for rheumatoid arthritis. Cochrane Database of Systematic Reviews. no. 2, p. CD000957.

Suarez-Almazor, M.E., Belseck, E., Shea, B., Wells, G. & Tugwell, P. (1998b). Sulfasalazine for rheumatoid arthritis. Cochrane Database of Systematic Reviews. no. 2, p. CD000958.

Tang, B.M., Guy, D.E., Nowson, C., Smith, C., Bensoussan, A., Bianchi, G., Czerwinski, E., Kenwright, A., Burdeska, A., Recker, R.R. & Felsenberg, D. (2012). Articles: Use of calcium or calcium in combination with vitamin D supplementation to prevent fractures and bone loss in people aged 50 years and older: a meta-analysis. *The Lancet.* **370** (9588), 657–66.

Tayar, J.H., Lopez-Olivo, M.A. & Suarez-Almazor, M.E. (2012). Febuxostat for treating chronic gout. Cochrane Database of Systematic Reviews. Issue 11. Art. No.: CD008653. DOI:10.1002/14651858.CD008653.pub2.

Toms, L., Derry, S., Moore, R.A. & McQuay, H.J. (2009). Single dose oral paracetamol (acetaminophen) with codeine for postoperative pain in adults. Cochrane Database of Systematic Reviews, Issue 1. Art. No.: CD001547. DOI: 10.1002/14651858.CD001547.pub2.

Toms, L., McQuay, H.J., Derry, S. & Moore, R.A. (2008). Single dose oral paracetamol (acetaminophen) for postoperative pain in adults. Cochrane Database of Systematic Reviews, Issue 4. Art. No.: CD004602. DOI: 10.1002/14651858.CD004602.pub2.

Towheed, T., Maxwell, L., Judd, M., Catton, M., Hochberg, M.C. & Wells, G.A. (2006). Acetaminophen for osteoarthritis. Cochrane Database of Systematic Reviews, Issue 1. Art. No.: CD004257. DOI: 10.1002/14651858. CD004257.pub2.

van den Berg, R., Baraliakos, X., Braun, J. & van der Heidje, D. (2012). First update of the current evidence for the management of ankylosing spondylitis with non-pharmacological treatment and non-biologic drugs: a systematic literature review for the ASAS/EULAR management recommendations in ankylosing spondylitis. *Rheumatology.* **51** (8), 1388–96.

van der Veen, M. J. & Bijlsma, J. W. (1993). The effect of methylprednisolone pulse therapy on methotrexate treatment of rheumatoid arthritis. *Clinical Rheumatology.* **12** (4), 500–505.

van Ojik, A.L., Jansen, P.A., Brouwers, J.R. & van Roon, E.N. (2012). Treatment of chronic pain in older people: evidence-based choice of strong-acting opioids. *Drugs and Aging.* **29** (8), 615–25.

von Keyserlingk., Hopkins, R., Anastasilakis, A., Toulis, K., Goeree, R., Tarride, J-E & Xie, F. (2011). Osteoporosis: Clinical efficacy and safety of denosumab in post-menopausal women with low bone mineral density and osteoporosis: A meta-analysis. *Seminars in Arthritis and Rheumatism.* **41**, 178–86.

Wells, G.A., Cranney, A., Peterson, J., Boucher, M., Shea, B., Welch, V., Coyle, D. & Tugwell, P. (2002). Risedronate for the primary and secondary prevention of osteoporotic fractures in post-menopausal women. Cochrane Database of Systematic Reviews, Issue 1. Art. No.: CD004523. DOI: 10.1002/14651858.CD004523. pub3

Watkins, P.B., Kaplowitz, N., Slattery, J.T., Colonese, C.R., Colucci, S.V., Stewart, P.W. & Harris, S.C. (2006). Aminotransferase elevations in healthy adults receiving 4 grams of acetaminophen daily: a randomized controlled trial. *The Journal of the American Medical Association.* **296**, 187–93.

Wells, G.A., Cranney, A., Peterson, J., Boucher, M., Shea, B., Welch, V., Coyle, D. & Tugwell, P. (2008a). Alendronate for the primary and secondary prevention of osteoporotic fractures in post-menopausal women. Cochrane Database of Systematic Reviews, Issue 1. Art. No.: CD001155. DOI: 10.1002/14651858.CD001155.pub2.

Wells, G.A., Cranney, A., Peterson, J., Boucher, M., Shea, B., Welch, V., Coyle, D. & Tugwell, P. (2008b). Etidronate for the primary and secondary prevention of osteoporotic fractures in post-menopausal women. Cochrane Database of Systematic Reviews. Issue 1. Art. No.: CD003376. DOI: 10.1002/14651858.CD003376.pub3.

Whiting, B., Holford, N. & Begg, E. (2002). Clinical Pharmacology. Principles and practice of drug therapy in medical education. *British Journal of Clinical Pharmacology.* **54** (1), 1.

Williams, H.J., Egger, M.J., Singer, J.Z., Willkens, R.F., Kalunian, K.C., Clegg, D.O., Skosey, J.L., Brooks, R.H., Alarcon, G.S. & Steen, V.D. (1994). Comparison of hydroxychloroquine and placebo in the treatment of the arthropathy of mild systemic lupus erythematosus. *Journal of Rheumatology.* **21** (8), 1457–62.

Wolff, R.F., Bala, M.M., Westwood, M., Kessels, A.G. & Kleijnen, J. (October 2010). 5% lidocaine-medicated plaster vs other relevant interventions and placebo for post-herpetic neuralgia (PHN): a systematic review. *Acta Neurologica Scandinavica.* doi: 10.1111/j.1600-0404.2010.01433.x.

Zhang, W., Doherty, M., Bardin, T., Pascual, E., Barskova, V., Conaghan, P., Gerster, J., Jacobs, J., Leeb, B., Liote, F., McCarthy, G., Netter, P., Nuki, G., Perez-Ruiz, F., Pignone, A., Pimentao, J., Punzi, L., Roddy, E., Uhlig, T. & Zimmermann-Gorska, I. (2006). EULAR evidence based recommendations for gout. Part II: Management. Report of a task force of the EULAR Standing Committee for International Clinical Studies Including Therapeutics (ESCISIT). *Annals of Rheumatic Disease.* **65** (10), 1312–24.

Index